The Stranger Comes At Sundown

Living And Dying
With Parkinson's Disease

Jane Kriete Awalt

ISBN 1-890689-33-5 (978-1-890689-33-9)

Library of Congress Cataloging-in-Publication Data

Awalt, Jane Kriete, 1924-
The stranger comes at sundown: living and dying with Parkinson's disease / Jane Kriete Awalt.
p. cm.
ISBN 1-890689-33-5 (978-1-890689-33-9)
ISBN 1-890689-59-9 (978-1-890689-59-9)
1. Awalt, Jane Kriete, 1924- 2. Awalt, Robert F.--Mental health
3. Parkinson's disease--Patients--United States--Biography. 4.
Caregivers--United States--Biography. 5. Caregivers--Family
relationships--United States. I. Title.
RC382.A93 2008
362.196'8330092--dc22
[B]
                                                    2008003043

The Stranger Comes At Sundown

Living And Dying
With Parkinson's Disease

Jane Kriete Awalt

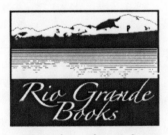

Los Ranchos, New Mexico

In Memoriam

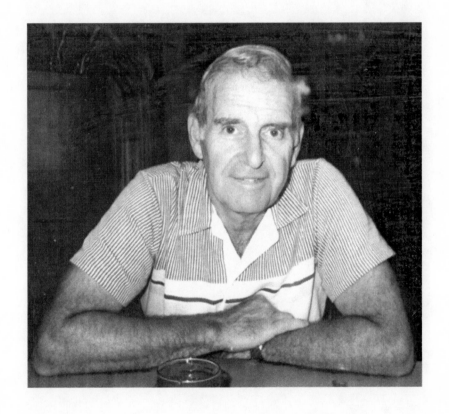

Robert F. Awalt
1924-2007

Contents

Preface ix

Introduction xi

The Changes, Physical & Mental 1

The Nursing Home Experience... 69

The Funeral and Its Preparations... 164

Things I Learned While Being a Caregiver 172

10 Tips for Family Caregivers... 176

Recommended Reading 176

PD Advocacy Organizations... 178

Professional Medical Associations 179

Parkinson Support Groups in Maryland 179

About the Author 185

Preface

*So slight and nearly imperceptible are the first
inroads of this malady, and so extremely slow its
progress, that it rarely happens, that the patient
can form any recollection of the precise period
of its commencement. The first symptoms perceived are, a slight sense of weakness, with a
proneness to trembling in some particular part,
sometimes in the head, but most commonly in
one of the hands and arms.*
                                    —James Parkinson, 1817

If you have been diagnosed with Parkinson's disease, you
will get lots of medical information on the various drug thera-
pies and medical procedures that may be available to you
for the treatment of this devastating disease. However, little
is available about the stages and the emotional side of Parkinson's. This book is a warm and tender journal on how one
man and his wife of 60 years dealt with the progression of
Parkinson's and coped with the daily changes brought about
by this illness.

Although he was diagnosed with Parkinson's in 1992, this
journal documents the progression that took control of Robert
F. Awalt between December 2005 and August 2007.

This journal is written especially for families and caregivers dealing with Parkinson's, but also for doctors and other medical professionals who need to understand what families living and dying with Parkinson's disease face.

Introduction

Parkinson's Disease

What Is Parkinson's Disease?

Parkinson's disease is a complex disorder. Parkinson's disease affects the way you move. It happens when there is a problem with certain nerve cells (neurons) in the brain. In normal circumstances these nerve cells produce an important chemical called dopamine. The dopamine chemical sends signals to the part of your brain that controls movement. Basically, dopamine allows your muscles to move smoothly and do what you want them to do. However, when you have Parkinson's disease, movement trouble comes when too many dopamine-producing neurons are lost. Then you no longer have enough dopamine, and you have trouble moving the way you want to move. The result is abnormal nerve firing patterns that produce impaired body movement.

It is estimated that at least half a million people in the United States have Parkinson's disease, and some estimates are much higher. In 2007 alone, it's estimated that another 50,000 people in this country will be diagnosed with the chronic, progressive movement disorder.

What Causes Parkinson's Disease?

No one knows for sure what makes these nerve cells break down. Age is one of the main risk factors for Parkinson's disease. People usually start to have symptoms between the ages of 50 and 60. Other possible factors are environmental agents such as poisons in the environment, midlife obesity, ongoing exposure to herbicides and pesticides, and drinking well water. Risk does seem to increase with age, so the disease is more typically seen in mid to late life. Interestingly, men seem to have a somewhat higher risk than do women. A family history of the disease may also increase risk, although there is not enough proof at this time to definitely say it's inherited. Abnormal genes seem to lead to Parkinson's disease in some people.

What Are The Symptoms?

The five main symptom categories of Parkinson's disease include:

1. Tremor, which means shaking or trembling. Tremor may affect your hands, arms, legs, or head.
2. Stiff muscles, rigid muscles in your limbs, stooped posture.
3. Slow movement, or shuffling walk.
4. Problems with balance, swallowing, or walking.
5. Trouble with thinking or memory.

Early-on signs and symptoms of Parkinson's disease may include a slight shaking in your hand or even one finger. Sometimes this hand tremor causes a back and forth rubbing of your thumb and forefinger known as pill-rolling. Tremor often starts in just one arm or leg or only on one side of the body. It could get worse as you are awake but not moving the affected arm or leg. The tremor may get better when you move the limb while you are asleep.

In time, Parkinson's may affect muscles throughout your body so it could even lead to trouble swallowing or constipation. In the later stages of the disease a person with Parkinson's may have a blank or fixed facial expression, trouble with speech, and many other problems.

Drug Treatments

Treatment for Parkinson's disease is highly individual and dependent on a case-by-case basis. Lifestyle changes such as a healthy diet and exercise may help. Some medications can help movement problems, but it does depend on how the disease is progressing. The main options to consider with your physician may include:

Dopamine replacers– Since its introduction in the 1960's Levadopa has been the main standard treatment. Nerve cells in the brain are capable of converting Levadopa to dopamine. Oftentimes it is prescribed in combination with Carbidopa (Sinemet). The drug Sinemet allows for the best dopamine benefit and reduces side effects of nausea and vomiting that can be associated with Levadopa alone. Many patients find this combination drug works for up to 15 years. There are also Dopamine agonists (Dopamine enhancers) that mimic dopamine's role in the brain; they are a little less potent than Levadopa but may have a longer lasting effect. In very advanced Parkinson's disease, deep brain stimulation that involves implanting a thin electrode in one of several locations in the brain is sometimes used. However, surgery isn't right for everyone. Things to consider before surgery are advanced age, problems with memory, or other serious medical problems which could make deep brain stimulation surgery risky.

Research Is Ongoing

Parkinson's disease continues to puzzle researchers, but scientists and physicians continue working on curing Parkinson's. Research efforts include cracking the protein code—in some families with the disease the breakdown of proteins has been impaired. There is a quest to discover how to selectively turn off production of the proteins, or at least to promote the breakdown of this protein. Another current research path is studying genomic pathways. Rather than focusing on a single gene that may be responsible for the disease, researchers are looking at a large cluster of related genes—a genomatic pathway—that seems to make some people more susceptible to Parkinson's disease.

Living With Loved Ones With Parkinson's Disease

Mrs. Jane Awalt's book on her life as a caregiver for her husband Bob Awalt and his battle with Parkinson's disease allows great insight into the disease and its affect on both the patient and the family and the spouse which is especially important for those half-million families affected by this progressive and relentless disease. This book will be especially useful for all of those affected by Parkinson's Disease. Her observations and tips will be especially useful to Parkinson's patients and their families.

Christa Arnold-Manning, Ph.D.
Senior Faculty
Dial Center for Written and Oral Communication
University of Florida
Niece of the beloved Bob Awalt

Sources

WebMd Healthwise (2007). Article link: http://www.webmd.com/parkinsons-disease/guide/parkinsons-disease-topic-overview.

http:/HealthLetter.MayoClinic.com (November 2007).

The Stranger Comes At Sundown
Living And Dying With Parkinson's Disease

The Changes, Physical & Mental

Today, 16 December, 2005, I have decided to keep a journal, of sorts, to record some of the changes, mentally and physically, in Bob Awalt, my husband of 58 years, who has Parkinson's disease which was diagnosed in 1992. This was the worst day I have experienced since we started down this path. For hours Bob thought I was his Aunt Marg and/or his mother. He couldn't figure out which person I was. I gave him many reminders, asked him who the mother of his children was, whom he married, and many other clues without success to break through his troubled mind.

This was the first time I really broke down and was in tears; but Bob did not seem to even notice how upset I was. I realize now the path this disease will take, and I will have no more surprises. You can imagine the worst and it is still not bad enough to explain how devastating this can make you feel to see someone who was so smart in everyway go downhill like this. I knew it would be bad but I had no idea there would be this feeling of helplessness for someone that means so much to me.

Aunt Marg Molz Schieswohl and her husband, Uncle George, lived in the second floor apartment of the home where my husband and his sister and brothers grew up. Aunt

Marg was almost like a second mother as she had no children of her own. She was always available to help out with the four boys and one girl of her sister Marie Molz Awalt.

When we went to dinner tonight, about 4pm, Bob recalled the confusion that he experienced earlier in the day. He remembered what happened and how mixed up he was but he said there was no way he could clear it up. He wanted to know who told me about it. He said it was not in the flesh, or looks, but a feeling that he had which he could not change even when he was looking straight at me. He ate well and seemed perfectly normal at dinner that we had with Bob's brother Jim and another couple. This is the first appearance of the Stranger in our house. He was trying to get into Bob's body and there was nothing Bob could do about it.

I shall call this journal, "The Stranger Comes At Sundown or Living & Dying With Parkinson's Disease." It is meant to help others suffering with Parkinson's disease, their families, and just to let them know they are not alone when these changes occur in their loved one.

Jane & Bob Awalt's Journal

Saturday, 17 December

I believe Bob had a pretty good night, judging from his bed, and he looks rested. Sometimes his mattress is moved four or five inches off of the springs. He had his breakfast and medication and is now completing a two hour nap. I am going to the Medical Supply store later to check out a power lift chair for him. He indicated that he wants to go with me so he can try it out. We will see if he can make it or not.

Saturday, 17 December — 12 Noon

This was a pretty good day after all. Bob did go and he tried out the power lift chairs, one of which we bought and it will be delivered the week after Christmas and before New Years day. We got home in time for him to have a nap for a half hour. Dinner was fine and there have been no problems. Bob had a nap after dinner for almost two hours.

Tonight Bob was speaking about how he felt. He said his mind was confused like it had blurred spots that he couldn't see through or make sense from. He also said that many times he couldn't make any distinction between Aunt Marg and me. He said again that even when he looks at me he can't tell the difference to know who is helping him. Anyway, his hair is cut and fingernails and toenails are cut and he has had a nice bath. Jim laughed and said I should hang out my shingle for cutting hair. Bob really does look good. I wish he felt as good as he looks. It is now 1am Sunday morning. I will turn in now.

Bob came in about 2am and asked me why his brother Jim was in his bed. (Jim lives in the same complex, but he has his own apartment.) He said Jim made some noise and awakened him. He just had another one of his bad dreams. But it took a lot of convincing him that Jim wasn't there. It is so strange that he can't look at the bed and not see Jim, and/or see the difference some of these dreams make.

Tuesday, 27 December

Today, our son Don made a wonderful suggestion to try to help his dad sleep most of the night rather than wake up off and on through out the night. He suggested that I put a small snack in his room for him to eat the first time he is awakened by the dreams and see if that helps. So, I put a plate with four small crackers with peanut butter on them and a glass half full of water. We will see how this works. It is now one thirty and he is still sleeping so I will also turn in for the night.

3

Sunday, 08 January

Well, I have stopped the snack in the middle of the night. Bob did eat the peanut butter and crackers but he still seems to have the awful dreams. Maybe we can think of another idea in the near future. It is very difficult for Bob to tell the difference between his dreams and reality.

Friday, 20 January

This was an especially difficult day for Bob. Early this morning he fell in the bathroom and was unable to awaken me by calling out to me. Bob's voice has become very soft and low making it almost impossible for me to hear him when he calls for help. I have given him a bell to shake and ring but of course it was in the bedroom. He must have been there a long time but he could not relate to anything to tell me how long. After much effort, we gave up trying to help him walk back to his bed. We decided it was safer for him to crawl back to his bed and thus eliminate the possibility of his falling again. He is suffering with a bad cold and it has sapped his strength completely. It also sounds like the cold is going down into his bronchial tubes. We used the wheel chair all day today. Fortunately I was able to wheel him to the table and he ate his dinner very well. Thank goodness.

Sunday, 21 January — 1am

I have been giving Bob hot tea, twice today, and the aspirin morning and evening, and he seems to feel better. He has also been walking some today. In fact, we didn't need to use the wheel chair at all today. He keeps telling me I don't realize how bad off he is. I let him know that I do, in fact, know exactly how ill he is but I try to keep our spirits up by not dwelling on it. I thought it might be a good time to cut his hair and he soaked his hands and I cut his fingernails for him. I do think it helped him feel better.

Bob seems so confused this evening plus he really has had a talking jag on, which is so unusual for him. He has been telling me that he just can't get it straight where we are at the present time. He can see water and beach area and it is like he has gone back in his memory to the times when we used to visit in Florida. He also spoke of how difficult it was to determine the difference between his mother and Aunt Marg when he looks at me. He says it is especially hard when I am doing something for him. This is so sad but it is not a shock like the first time this subject came up. I will finish up and go to bed shortly.

Tuesday, 28 February

Today Bob had another very bad fall, he was going from the sunroom into my bedroom, where he was going to rest on the twin bed and watch TV. Within a minute or so the paramedics were here and at that time they were able to help him regain consciousness. Six paramedics came and were very good with Bob. They bandaged his hand, which was cut, took all of his vital signs, which were OK and returned two more times to check on him. He was up most of last night and slept most of today and I was able to get a good nap also, which was greatly needed. His walking is very bad and we used the wheel chair in the apartment and it was a big help. He still sees people in the bedroom and it is mostly our daughter Barbe and our son Don or his mother and Aunt Marg. These hallucinations are very real to Bob and are a side effect of Parkinson's disease and also the Sinemet which treats the symptoms of the disease.

Wednesday, 01 March

Things were a little better tonight. However, Bob was still a little confused as to where he was and what happened yesterday. He had a good dinner of crab cake, mashed potatoes, peas, milk, and two pieces of chocolate cream pie that we got in a carry-out order. He seemed to enjoy this meal very much. I think he is weaker than he was and this gets worse at night. We used the wheel chair in the apartment again and this saves a lot of wear and tear on him. I also had him soak his hands where the cuts are and I cut his fingernails. I like to keep them short so he doesn't scratch himself in his sleep. He has some wild dreams sometimes and it is hard to tell what he will do. The Stranger still tries to get into Bob's body, which he knows, but he is unable to do anything about it.

Monday, 06 March

Well, we had a pretty bad night, that is to say, not much sleep. We have had to have two bedrooms because the dreams Bob has are too violent. He thrashes about and I would not get any sleep. I stayed up until about 2am, thinking that would be about the first time Bob usually awakens with his bad dreams. I heard a noise in his room, not too loud, but I knew he had fallen. I went in and sure enough he was down on the floor.

The nightmares awaken him and he decides he has to go to the bathroom. He has a urinal in his bedroom but he takes it in to the bathroom to use.

His legs are like jelly so he has to crawl back to his bed and then he has a terrible time trying to get up onto the bed. We struggled for forty-five minutes and at 2:15am, we finally managed to have him in bed and comfortable

I got him all tucked into bed, return to my bed and just about get to sleep and I hear the thump again. I run into his bedroom and there he is down on the floor again. This was about 3:30am. We go through the same routine again, he crawls to his bed and after much effort we finally get him back in bed. No injuries from these two falls but we are both exhausted from working to get Bob back in bed and settled for the rest of the night.

Today, I think he felt a little better, although he couldn't walk much better. Now he is sitting in his wheelchair shaving for the first time since the fall on Tuesday and his face looks very good. He also made out well today by taking a shower, rather than the tub bath. The tub bath does make his legs feel good but we were afraid he might not be able to pull up to get out of the tub. Now, we will see what happens tonight and I hope it is lots of sleep for both of us.

Monday, 13 March

Well, surprise of all surprises. I was awakened this morning by the sound of voices talking, which I thought were the people picking up the trash in the hall. As I listened the voices became louder and sounded like they were coming from inside our apartment. This is exactly where they were coming from, in our living room. I jumped out of bed and walked into the living room, still in my nightgown. There was a security man, with Bob in a wheelchair. Bob had opened the door of the apartment, walked down the long hall to the reception room and there he sat speaking with the lady who delivers the papers. She was the one who called security people to come and help Bob. He sat there with his pajama top on, his bathrobe over that and nothing else. He had no pajama pants on, nor did he have any slippers or shoes on.

He later said he was surprised that he wasn't arrested for doing this. Although he knew what he did, he couldn't explain why. He said at the time it just didn't matter to him. He was unable to analyze the situation.

Tonight Bob's mind is still clouded over, as he calls it. He is still confused as to who I am. When he is tired and about an hour before he goes to bed seems to be the worst time for him. He couldn't understand why Jim wasn't with us anymore. Jim never did live with us. He asked many unusual questions about our life here in our nice apartment. The fact that we have lived here for six and one half years has escaped his memory completely. This seems to be the time the Stranger enters Bob's mind and body, which he is aware of but he has no control over this Stranger.

Tuesday, 14 March

We both had a good sleep last night for the first time in a very long time. This was seven hours of uninterrupted sleep. Bob looked better today and I felt so much better. I hope this continues. I have started giving Bob one Tylenol PM before bedtime and it really worked last night. Of course, the "overnight brief" didn't work completely and the sheets were also wet but I quickly changed the bed and thought this was a small price to pay for such a good night's sleep. I do hope this continues as I continue to use the Tylenol PM. He even walked to the dining room for dinner tonight. This dining room is the one that is at the extreme end of the complex of buildings on our campus. I will turn in now and we will see what happens tomorrow.

Thursday, 16 March

This was one of those nights that the Tylenol PM didn't work at all. Bob was awake and up every two hours and his mind was very cloudy (as he calls it.) He urinated on the floor and rugs when he just couldn't make it in time to the bathroom plus pushing down the "overnight brief" which has been so helpful in keeping him and the bed dry.

He still seems to be so confused about 8pm each evening. I still think it is because he is tired and ready for bed. Yet, if he goes to bed this early, he will be awake most of the night. It is also difficult for him to get interested in television. What a shame!!! The Stranger seems to know exactly when to get into Bob's mind and body and he continues to make his appearance about the same time in the evening.

Saturday, 18 March

Last night was better with only one interruption about 6am and then we both went back to bed. What a difference it makes to have a reasonably good night's sleep. Earlier Bob promised to stay put and watch television or nap while I went up to the store, which he did. The food store is about ten minutes away. In fact, he was sound asleep when I returned

Sunday, March 19

Last night was terrible. Bob said he didn't know how much more he could stand of this disease. He used up all of the "overnight briefs" and I had to try a different kind, which were awful. Urine was everywhere, bed, and floor and night clothes. I had also given him two of the Tylenol PM tablets to help him sleep, which didn't work at all. I did go to the store again, especially to get the fresh Tylenol PM, and got home and the box was not in my package. I called the store and they said they would replace them. However, it is the inconvenience of another trip to the store. I hope they work!

Monday, 20 March

We both had six and one half hours sleep last night. The new brief didn't work so I am going to take the rest of the package back to the store today sometime.

I have located where the others are being sold, under a different name, and just up the road at Wal-Mart store. So, I will drive up there when Bob is taking a nap.

I want to reassure our children, and Jim, when I think we need help I will look into it. So far, there is nothing going on that I can't handle and I am glad to take care of and help Bob. If I can keep him dry at night, the rest of what I do is a piece of cake, or Boston cream pie, which is a favorite of Bob's.

Bob is shaving now, getting ready for his bath. He has had a great haircut and will be all ready for the special "reservation-only" dinner tomorrow night. I have all of the bed clothes in the washing machine, great having washer and dryer in the apt. It is wonderful to get a good night's sleep. It makes such a difference in how I feel the next day. I can make out fine if I get a good night's sleep a few nights a week.

I realize it is hard for our children to have to watch and hear all of the history of their father's last illness. I believe a lot of Bob's problems now, especially at night, might have more to do with our aging than his Parkinson's disease. We are not spring chickens anymore. I tell the children they have seen the best of us and now there is a different side to see.

I ask our children not to worry too much. They should be glad and thankful that we are here, in a nice apartment and we are settled. I would not want to have to move now.

Just an update on today. Bob finished shaving, did a great job, finished his bath and while he took a nap, I went up to Wal-Mart and got exactly the type of "special brief," which I hope will be the solution to his nighttime problem of not staying dry. He still had not awakened by the time I returned home.

Tonight, Jim has his meeting and dinner at St. Joseph's Church so we are on our own. Instead of carry-out we are having dinner with another couple whom we have not eaten with in a long time. I actually think Bob is looking forward to it. I will take him in the wheelchair so he doesn't get too tired going to dinner. Maybe he will push the chair home afterwards so he can get a little exercise.

It has been a good day so far for Bob to shave, bathe and dress without being so tired that he had to rest. This time, when he shaved, he didn't even use the electric razor. He really did a great job. Good old sleep makes a big difference. Some days he is just too weak to shave.

Tuesday, 21 March

Life is getting back to normal. We slept until 5:30 and went back to bed until 8:30. This is a good thing!!! Bob had his medication and has gone back for a short nap. (Ha-ha) His bed is dry, as he is, so I know the brief has worked. Maybe we will have another good day.

I am going to make Jim a bib, like Bob's, for him to use in his apartment. I doubt if he uses it in the dining room. The couple last night thought it was a great idea making the bib out of towels. The wife said she would love to have one like it. I told her I would be glad to make her one. She looked so surprised that I don't know if she was just kidding, about wanting one, or that I would make her one. I can't figure people out anymore.

We did have a good time at the Special Dinner, and it was so good. Crab soup was first and then the main entry was rockfish stuffed with seafood, shrimp, crab etc and baked Alaska for dessert. It was delicious but too much food. Bob didn't want to go at the last minute but he did enjoy every bit of it. He also drank a small glass of wine. He is asleep now. It was a good time with friends whom we usually eat with at these special dinners.

Wednesday, 22 March

This was another good night with six and one half hours of uninterrupted sleep. It is great!!! I am so glad everything is working out for Bob. The "special briefs" worked perfectly. The bed, floor, and Bob were completely dry. This makes him feel so much better than having accidents all over the place when he can't get to the bathroom in time. Life is wonderful.

Today started off really good after having a good night's sleep. We decided to go to the McCormick shareholders meeting at Hunt Valley. We made out fine, Bob walked in fine and seemed to enjoy the meeting. When we left and got out of the main room he couldn't walk. It was like his legs were jelly. I took one arm and he held on to a lady's walker as she also moved slowly along.

When we got to the reception area, Bob sat on the edge of one of the tables. The people were so kind to him, one ran and got him a glass of water, which he needed for his medication. They also sent for the man who is head of security for McCormick, who was wonderful to Bob. He got him a chair, two poles with a rope, and roped his area off so no one could get near him.

We were in the middle of eleven hundred and forty people, so they announced. After a short while, the medication worked and security was called for a wheelchair. Bob was wheeled to the main entrance of the Marriott until I got the car. This man was wonderful with Bob.

This afternoon I emailed a letter to the Customer Service of McCormick telling them that I thought the kindness of security was well beyond the call of duty. I am sure he was late for the special luncheon that they have for their executive people but he was not rushed one bit.

If we go next year, I will take the wheelchair in the trunk of the car. In fact, I may try taking him to Towson one day. He will get some air and have a nice change. I told him this tonight and he suggested going to Whole Foods. WOW! I said to him. Yes, we will. He never did like Towson much. There has been too much trouble there.

I keep telling him that it isn't right for him to stay in the apartment all day and just go to the dining room to eat in the evening. So, if we have a good night's sleep tonight, we will not have to nap in the daytime and who knows, maybe we will be able to go out for a ride.

Monday 27 March

This day didn't start off too badly but as it went on, it became worse and worse. Bob wanted to ride to Sam's Club with me as I needed just a few things, one of which was my prescription for blood pressure. He was so miserable in the store and I had so much trouble getting him to the car that I was completely distracted and left my medication in the cart. I called the store, when I realized, and someone had found it and turned it in to them. I will go and pick it up tomorrow. I was going to stop and get "carry-out" for our dinner tonight, instead of going to the dining room, but we were too late. You must get the "carry-out" between 2pm and 3pm, therefore we went to the dining room later. We had one of his favorite dishes tonight but he ate very little. Naturally I pushed him over to the dining room in his wheelchair that he stayed in to sit at the table.

When we arrived home, Bob had to go the bathroom so I suggested he use the stairs and I would use the elevator, as I had a cart with the things from the store. When I got off the elevator, he was nowhere in sight and I spent a half hour, with a security guard, looking for him. He had wandered into the reception room and some of the cleaning ladies had showed him where the men's room was and then he got lost on the wrong floor. We finally found him but it certainly upset him. There is definitely some change in his speech tonight. I could hardly understand him. The Stranger is entering his body earlier now but Bob still has no control over him even though Bob knows he has returned to his body.

I have spent from seven o'clock tonight until eleven trying to get him comfortable in bed. Finally we managed to get him in. He tries so hard to help but he is just unable to help at all. I hope tomorrow is better for him. I finally gave him some warm milk with some Old Granddad in it. He has never been a drinker and this bottle is left over from his retirement in 1986. I am not sure if I will go to bed or stay up, and nap tomorrow when he does, to make sure he is alright.

Tuesday, 28 March

Wow! What a night. I am glad I decided to stay up as I had the virus all night long. I was so glad the Tylenol PM was helping Bob to sleep. I just felt like I wanted to sleep away the day, which we both did. We had a light meal—soup, bread and a cup of tea. Bob just had an orange, cut up and some grapes. Bob protested, but I got it down him. I have been watching him closely so he doesn't dehydrate. His cold seems better but he is a mess. I have an appointment tomorrow for him to see the doctor. I just don't like the way he is acting or looks. I also think he may have a little blood in his urine.

I do feel better, just uneasy on my feet, which I think is a little weakness. I do not think I can take care of him much longer. He is so helpless and I do not have much strength to help him. We spent more than an hour tonight just to get him from the wheelchair into his bed. There must be a better way to help him.

Wednesday, March 29 —3:15am

Bob got out of bed, of course his legs won't hold him, down he went, and we have been one half hour trying to get him to crawl back and then get him in bed. What a job! I hope I can get him to the medical center which at this point I doubt.

Yes, I was able to get Bob to the Medical Center. The doctor thought at first that Bob may have had a heart attack. However, when the blood work was returned all was okay and it did not indicate there were the particles in Bob's blood that the heart throws off, when one has a heart attack.

The doctor authorized Bob to have a medication such as Pepsid Complete if necessary. Bob was also given nitroglycerin, which was used once but I think the problem cleared up on its own. I really believe there must have been something to upset Bob's diet that caused this temporary discomfort.

Friday, 07 April

Well, today was another one of those with Bob having strange ideas about who I am. He just couldn't get it straight that I was Jane, his wife. He asked me if people around here could recognize me and, if so, how did they know me. I tried to explain I was his wife of almost 59 years in June. He also asked me if I had nursing experience. After I told him that taking care of him was my only nursing experience, he told me his sister was a nurse. He also thought she had moved out West. I immediately told him I thought he was thinking of his daughter, Barbe, who had moved out to Albuquerque, New Mexico. He then agreed that was who he was thinking of who moved away.

By the time Bob went to bed tonight at eleven o'clock his mind seemed to clear and he had no more of the strange questions. The Tylenol PM does not seem to work every night so tonight I gave him two aspirin and they seemed to help the pain in his legs. I hope they help him sleep through the night.

Saturday, 08 April

The aspirin worked very well last night. We each had six hours of uninterrupted sleep, which was wonderful. However, in the morning Bob was soaking wet as was his bed. I do not understand why the "all-night" briefs do not work to keep him dry. I use three on him at night and still they do not work to keep him dry. The one good thing is that Bob does not get out of bed to walk to the bathroom.

The daytime seems to be no problem with him using a urinal, which he uses every two hours. I am glad the doctor did the blood work testing his PSA because I thought there could be a problem there. The 2.8 reading seems to be in line for a normal situation.

His elimination is getting very regular now, every day about

3:30 when we are getting ready to go and eat in the dining room he has the urge to go to the bathroom. Of course he has trouble getting adjusted to the toilet seat arrangement, which is used now to raise the toilet seat so he doesn't have to sit so low as on the regular toilet seat. I think this is finally getting a little easier for him. The new seat does have a strong handle bar on each side to assist him in standing from the sitting position.

Tonight I tried rubbing oil on his legs to see if it would help the pain he seems to suffer with every night. I can't understand why his legs don't bother him in the daytime. The pain seems to start every night, after dinner, at about eight o'clock. When he goes to bed the pain seems to disappear and his legs don't bother him at all. His legs certainly do not support him now. He can walk a few steps but then his feet freeze to the floor.

Bob had his two aspirin again tonight and we will see if they work well again. It will be good to have two nights in a row of uninterrupted sleep. Since it is now 2am, I will turn in and hope I can get to sleep right away.

Wednesday, 12 April

Many changes are taking place in Bob's mind at this time. First of all, he can hardly focus to see anything. This can be due to the macular degeneration and/or the cataracts or probably both. This has taken the last pleasure he had, of watching the TV. He does seem to listen to the news but doesn't pay much attention to anything else on the TV. He continues to tell me how difficult it is for him to concentrate that I am aware of since he stopped reading the newspaper and some magazines that he formerly enjoyed.

Bob still cannot get used to using the toilet with the extension on it. If he doesn't use a urinal he will urinate all over the bathroom floor. The same thing happens when he has an elimination. The muscles in that lower area like all of his muscles barely work right now. This has been very distressing for him to accept that when he has an elimination, if he isn't sitting on the toilet correctly, he goes all over everything, including himself, the toilet and sometimes the floor. This usually makes an awful mess so I just ask him to get into the shower, which he does gladly.

Sometimes he has to take a shower twice a day to stay clean and free of odor. He wears three sets of special briefs at night and they worked very well last night. In fact, he slept until eight o'clock this morning, which was a nice change.

Once again, I must say how glad I am that we have a big washer and dryer in our apartment. We are both glad to be settled in now. When Bob realizes the work that was left behind at our house, when we owned property, it is especially gratifying. I can concentrate on helping Bob now rather than help take care of property, which would be impossible now, at our ages, and Bob's disease.

Bob is talking a lot now about "He just can't take much more of this disease." When he told me this tonight I asked him if he was ready to call it quits. He responded that he was if he couldn't get any better. He said, "This is a terrible way to live." I told him again how lucky we had been up to now and that we had almost 59 years of marriage that was good. Also, for most of those years we have been very healthy. His mind was clearer tonight when he was talking along these lines. He did not question who I was or when we moved to the apartment or some of the other questions that have been so puzzling. The Stranger was absent this evening and therefore we were able to talk together without interruptions from him.

Naturally, I don't know how near the end is for Bob. This is such a sad time leading up to the time when he is free of pain and discomfort. I hope he has a peaceful end because he has suffered so this last year. It might not be so bad if his mind was not clear most of the time and he did not realize what changes were happening to him. His battle with the Stranger is ongoing and will be Bob's major problem for the future, I am afraid.

Thursday, 13 April

Last night was miserable for both of us. Nothing worked to help Bob sleep. I tried the two aspirin, and a small glass of wine, without success. Today was not much better. Bob was very weak all day, would not eat and stayed in bed most of the day. One bright spot was Jim stopping over for a short visit, which Bob liked very much. Tonight he did eat a very good dinner so the muscles in his throat are still working. I was worried about them when he wouldn't eat all day.

It is now eleven o'clock and Bob is in bed and I am on my way to bed. We are both hopeful of getting a good night's sleep tonight. I hope we are not disappointed. The Social Worker called up today for an appointment to come and visit and talk. So, I made one with her for next Thursday.

I keep telling people I am doing what I want and when it gets too much I will get some help in the home. Until then, I hope everyone will stop suggesting that I need some help.

Friday, 14 April

What a night! From 6pm to 10pm I have been trying to keep Bob awake so he will sleep through the night. What a job! He has asked me all sorts of strange questions and I have tried to answer him.

Every five minutes he would ask me how much longer until bed time. He just can't understand how it works that if you nap right before bedtime there is no way you will go right off to sleep and continue to sleep through the night.

Friday, 05 May

We finally have the procedure to work right, at night, for

keeping Bob and the bed dry. I use three different types of briefs from the package that advertises they are for "night and/or day" usage. None of these work by themselves but together they work fine. Bob finally understands that he is not to get up during the night to go to the bathroom. One type of brief is a slip-on, with two elastic bands that button into the slip-on. Over this goes a large wrap-around brief that has three closures, like Velcro, on each side. Over this goes a regular night or day brief that holds all in place. Then over all three of these goes a pair of regular underwear shorts to keep everything in place and make a really snug fit.

Bob's walking has gotten so bad that he is crawling a lot of the time to get to a chair or the bed, or for a nap in the afternoon. His legs are just like jelly and his knees sound like bones cracking together. He could hardly stand in the bathroom this evening to shave.

Saturday, 06 May

Tomorrow is Sunday so we will get a "carry-out" dinner. Jim will eat with his friend and get some interesting conversation, as he says. Bob is always disappointed when Jim decides he wants to go to the brunch early on Sunday. However, this is a good change for Jim and Bob does like a "carry-out" meal that we can eat in the apartment.

I am still giving Bob two aspirin about a half an hour before he goes to bed at night. This really seems to help him. He also gets two aspirin about a half hour before we go to the dining room in the evening and this seems to help the pain in his legs so that he can eat his dinner in peace. This has been a big help. In between is the time he takes his Sinemet for the Parkinson's disease. He now gets this medication every two hours beginning at 8am.

Bob still speaks of the people that he thinks he sees standing around the apartment. Some of them, he will recognize and others he does not. He sees our daughter, Barbe, a lot. He rarely sees our son, Don. Most of the time it seems to be his mother and Aunt Marg. Many times in the evening he still confuses me with them. Sometimes he will ask me if I am going to leave at night and what time will I leave. The other night when we were talking of how we happened to move into the apartment and when we sold our house there was some mention of money. Out of a clear blue sky, he said he thought Jane took care of all of the money expenses. I asked him who he thought I was and he looked confused. When I told him I was Jane, his wife, he replied that sometimes he gets me mixed up with others.

Saturday, 13 May

Well, this was a most peculiar night speaking with Bob. He really gave me the third degree about who I was. Did I have nurse's training? What was my maiden name and who my parents were, especially my father's name? He just did not believe me when I told him my maiden name was Kriete. He said I was playing tricks on him.

His mind was so cloudy that he said he could not believe I was Jane, his wife. Many times he asked me what my maiden name was. Over and over again, this was repeated for more than one hour. Finally, he said the whole thing upset him and he would have to forget it for the night.

Sunday, May 14

Once again I was awakened, about 5am, with two loud bumps on the floor, or so it sounded. I got up and went into see how Bob was doing. There he was on the floor, in his bedroom, unable to stand and get up. I worked with him and he was finally able to get back up on his bed. Although his hands were warm, he was very cold. He seems to get so cold on the inside of his body even though he feels warm to touch.

I put another blanket on him and he drifted off to sleep before I left his room.

Fortunately, the special briefs still are working well at night. The bed was dry, as he was. This helps to keep him more comfortable. In the kitchen, under the table, the part of the kitchen that is the sunroom is a lovely oriental rug. Bob quickly urinated on the rug. I guess it won't be long before all of the beds, rugs and floors will have been christened in this manner. I try hard to keep him off of my bed because he has two beds that he alternates sleeping and napping on. I keep plastic on his bed for sleeping at night but I guess that will not last too long.

Dinner was good, as Bob did eat well. I will worry when he doesn't eat at all. Don came over, which was nice, and Jim joined us for dinner and this was a nice affair. I believe with everything considered Bob had a pretty good day.

Monday, 15 May

Bob again had the cloud over his mind, as he calls it. He just can't keep in his mind who I am and if there are two people who come in to care for him. He questioned me again tonight and I finally gave up. He still thinks these two people come to work in two different shifts. When he hugged and kissed me goodnight, he was in his bed, I asked him if he knew who I was. His answer was in the negative and I asked him if he kissed everyone. He laughed and said no. He finally said he thought I was Mary, his mother. I smiled and told him to close his eyes and go to sleep and in the morning we would talk about it again. It must be because he is tired at night that he seems so confused about who I am or what is happening when the Stranger is trying to enter his mind and body.

I guess he will have to start wearing the nighttime briefs in the daytime now. Tonight, he had an accident on the guest room bed and wet a large area in the center of the mattress.

I am so glad I have not bought the new mattresses. I will have to get a large piece of plastic for this bed like I use on his sleeping bed. He just naps on the single bed in the guest room. He sleeps on a double bed in his room at night. We will now see what happens tomorrow.

Tuesday, 16 May

The questions did flow this evening. Bob knew his mind was clouded over. It was like he couldn't do anything right. He urinated on the bed again, and on the floor beside the bed. He kept asking where the other worker was and when did she come to work. We were both glad when bedtime rolled around. It appears the time is becoming earlier, in the day, when the Stranger begins to make his appearance in Bob's mind and body.

Wednesday, 17 May

We both had a very good night, after all of the problems last night. Bob slept through the night until 7am and then went back to bed until 9am. He was dry and everything in his bed was dry. What a big help. He had his shower early and shaved and was all spruced up when Don came over bringing roast beef sandwiches with potato salad. Don was so glad to see him eat well and enjoy his food. So far this is not a problem. We had a nice visit and Bob took his nap while I went to the food store, which is up the road a short distance. It was so good to have this "Peace of Mind" while shopping. When I returned home Bob was still asleep and Don left and I was able to take a much needed short nap.

Bob's mind was clouded again tonight. He asked many of the same questions over and over again. He can't understand the situation of where we now live and why we sold our house. After much discussion I suggested we continue this conversation in the morning. Bob agreed because he said he could not understand it tonight. So be it! This Stranger is working overtime trying to destroy Bob's mind and body.

Friday, 19 May

We had a few good surprises today. First of all, Bob remembered, on his own, how to use the urinal, which he used frequently with success. He really had a very good day today, almost what I would call "a normal day".

Then, after he was all shaved, washed and completely dressed to go to the dining room, he remarked that his pants were wet. Sure enough he had an accident and urinated, in his pants, without the special protective briefs on, and everything had to be changed. Yes, you can bet he has the special protective briefs back on. He has been wearing them mostly at night. I guess we won't take chances anymore.

Dinner was uneventful except for the fact that he pushed his wheelchair all the way to the dining room, which is on the extreme end of where we live on campus. He walked very well, ate well, rode part of the way back home, and walked about a third of the way back home. He really had good exercise this evening, which tired him out, and he has taken a nice long nap. Now we will see what surprises tonight will bring after several nights of sleeping all the way through, which has been great. Bob was able to keep the Stranger out of his mind and body this time, for a change.

Monday, May 22

Today started off terribly with Bob calling me to get up at four fifteen this morning. Bob was just walking around with his red flashlight in his hand, shining it all around at the window and acting like he was in a trance. He really hollered at me not to take his flashlight from him and he actually fought me so that I could not take it. Finally, when I got him in bed, I got the flashlight out of his hand and put it in the bed next to his pillow. This satisfied him and we both went back to sleep.

This was one awful night and I don't think I could get back to sleep until almost seven o'clock in the morning. The Stranger is still trying to win. He did succeed in winning a battle but he has not won the war as yet. Bob is still having some quality time although it is not often.

Tonight Bob expressed how he felt by saying that he felt like his body was upside down. He said it was very strange. He did not seem to have the cloud over his brain; but he just wanted to go to bed early, which he did, and we will see how he sleeps. It was not a good day and he was very glad we decided to get "carry-out" instead of going to the dining room for dinner. Tomorrow, Don and his wife Kathy and Barbe will be here for a visit. Barbe will just be here two days from Albuquerque but I think it will be long enough for her to see how much her dad's health has failed. I am hoping he will have a good day and enjoy her visit.

Thursday, 25 May

I solved the flashlight problem by removing one of the batteries and reversing it so the flashlight would not come on. I know that Bob is smart enough that if he picked up the flashlight without the batteries, he would know instantly that I removed the batteries. So far, it has worked or else this particular effort, on his part, is completely forgotten.

We had a nice visit with Barbe, here from Albuquerque, for the two days. Things were pretty good during the daytime visits. It was especially nice the night that Don, Kathy, Jim and Barbe were all here. Don brought in delicious crab cake sandwiches, and wine, Barbe brought in a delicious carrot cake. I made cole slaw, got some beer, and we really had a dinner party. Bob ate very well and looked like he enjoyed the food and the family gathering very much.

After everyone left Bob was really upset and kept talking about how could anybody say "How good he looked" when he felt so bad. I explained they could not see inside to see how he felt. They were only looking at him on the outside. Finally, he went to bed, he slept very well, which was a blessing because I was very tired.

Bob has continued to speak of how good the family thought he looked everyday since they were here visiting and even this morning when we talked about Barbe flying home from Baltimore. Maybe he will forget how good his children thought he looked and stop talking about it. He continues to tell me that I don't know how bad off he really is. I do know how miserable he feels most of the time but I try not to dwell on it when I am with him because I think it will make him feel worse.

Today we have spent about every half hour going into the bathroom to check and see if Bob could have his elimination, without success. He gets like this frequently and we just have to work with it. I must say our nights continue to be much better, bed dry, Bob dry, and we both get about five or six hours sleep. What a relief! I just wish he could feel better during the daytime.

We got carry-out for our dinner tonight as Bob absolutely refused to go to the dining room because he felt so miserable. He really couldn't eat so I spoon-fed him his entire meal, which he seemed to like, once he got it down.

Bob still can't get the hang of sitting on the toilet seat. Instead he urinates all over the floor, which makes an awful mess. I will go in now and scrub the floor up and put the towels that he tried to wipe up the floor with, in the wash. He tries so hard but sometimes I wish he wouldn't.

Wednesday, May 31

This evening was a little better than most nights. He did not have the cloud hanging over his mind like he usually does.

He said for three weeks he thought I was two people and he could not tell the difference between his mother, Aunt Marg or me. He said he does not have that feeling now. He still has so much trouble using the urinal and gets so upset when I try to tell him what to do. He said it is easier just to urinate on the floor. He does not retain any direction now and gets upset when I tell him how to do anything. Later he said he was sorry, that he didn't want to be nasty, but sometimes he just couldn't help himself. He has a bad habit of blaming me for anything that goes wrong with him. I tried to explain that it is his Parkinson's disease that causes these different things to happen and he can not blame anyone. It is just an accident of Mother Nature that has caused this disease to develop. No one knows why or how it happens. It is difficult for him to understand but he did apologize which made me feel awful. I do wish there was more I could do to help him.

I have pleaded with Bob to stay in bed at night. Last night he walked all around, fell twice on his knees, and kept coming in to awaken me to see if I was alright. He said he heard someone screaming for help. I didn't hear any sound so I am pretty sure he was dreaming. Most times these dreams are so real it is hard to convince him that it is really a dream. Many times he is not fully awake himself. However, tonight, I told him I really needed sleep. He naps through the day, which I can't always take the time to do. I hope he remembers.

Thursday, 01 June

We had a very successful night with each of us getting eight hours sleep. Bob just had a complete elimination so I hope he will have a much better day. My side is still very painful where I hurt it the other night trying to help Bob get up. Usually, he is dead weight and it really takes a lot of effort. I will have to be very careful in the future. I have one of the "Heat Strips" on the area but the skin gets damp and the strip will not stick. I put an Ace bandage around my body, over the heat strip, to keep it in place. I have the Ace bandage very loose and it does seem to do the job of keeping the heat strip in place. I took the two aspirin and hope to get some relief soon. I plan on soaking in the tub later and it usually helps. Here's looking forward to a better day.

Monday, 05 June

The routine has remained the same every day now. I guess all Bob's natural functions are seriously handicapped. The urination and the complete elimination ability have become unpredictable now with Bob. It must be the muscles in the lower area that are involved. But what a mess! His underwear, the bed sheet, where he watches TV, the chair, the flannel throw on the bed all messed up and wet. I must say again and again that I am glad to have such a good washer and dryer.

Bob continues to have the cloud over his mind every evening. I am sure this will always be the cause of his frustration. He knows this happens and he is totally miserable with it. However, he cannot do anything to stop it from happening. Nights are about the same with giving us five or six hours sleep. I hope this continues because it is better than no sleep. I hope and pray the Stranger does not continue to dictate Bob's actions since there is no solution to this problem.

Tuesday, 06 June

Last night was another one of those terrible nights with Bob walking the floor beginning at 4am constantly until we finally got up about eight o'clock. He was wet as well as his bed, soaked clear through. He takes off his special briefs and that leaves him with no protection if he has an accident in bed. It has been a day in which Bob could not eat much, feeling sick as he ate, but did not actually get sick. This is the same pattern that happened last night. He just couldn't eat very much although he still feels very weak. I have spoon-fed him, the little he did eat, both last night and today.

Tonight at dinner, Bob did eat better but it took much coaxing and encouragement for him to get his food down. His legs hurt him badly and when they do this pain interferes with everything including eating.

Bob still has confusion in the bathroom and can't seem to remember how to flush the toilet. He worries about this and keeps complaining that something is wrong with the toilet. I explained to him that nothing is wrong with the toilet but his muscles don't work correctly for him. All of the muscles are involved with Parkinson's disease and he just can't understand this. I keep demonstrating how the toilet flushes but he still thinks something is wrong with the toilet. It is so difficult to compete with the Stranger when he is trying to enter Bob's mind and body that we both become frustrated.

I hope he has a good night of sleep. I have given him the two aspirin with the stool softener and I hope they work. I am really tired and would love to have a good night's sleep of seven or eight hours sleep but I won't count on it.

Wednesday, 07 June

Boy, what a difference a day can make. In the first place, we both had eight hours of good sleep.

As the day proceeded, Bob felt worse and worse. He really wanted to get "carry-out" and not go to the dining room. He did consent to a nice long bath, to soak his legs, and seemed to feel much better when he finished. We went to dinner, Bob using the wheelchair, and then he got out, of the wheelchair, to sit at the table. He hardly made it to the chair at the table, which was only one step away. However, he ate his dinner like he hadn't eaten in a week. He said later he really enjoyed his dinner. He ate soup, chopped steak with mushrooms, mashed potatoes with gravy, spinach, ice cream and another dessert. WOW! Like I said he really enjoyed his dinner. Now, we will see what happens tonight.

Thursday, 08 June

Today was another bad day for Bob. He was unable to have his elimination and this always seems to set him off in another direction. This evening he had a short nap and when he awakened he was really confused. Once again he thought there were two people taking care of him and this apartment. He also saw two people that he wondered why they were here. He wasn't sure but he thought they were his mother and Aunt Marg. He asked me if I ever met his mother and how did I meet her. He also asked me how we met. Keep in mind we have been married for almost 59 years and visited his parents regularly when they were alive. He just couldn't seem to grasp the idea that there is only his wife here with him now. Maybe later on there will be others, to help take care of him, but they will only add to his confusion.

Bob still felt so bad at bedtime that he had a really rough time getting ready for bed. Since he couldn't walk very well he had to crawl into the bathroom and when it was time to use the water pick, he had to stay on his knees. He was unable to have his teeth brushed tonight so at least the water pick gets any food that is in between his teeth. He has such beautiful teeth. The disease is a slow moving disease, in most cases, but it is certainly making Bob incapacitated now.

Sunday, 11 June

Yesterday is a day that we will remember for a long time. It started about 3pm when Bob felt so bad that he did not want to go to dinner. It was too late to get "carry-out" so I encouraged him to shave and get ready to go to dinner. He finished his bath and I really thought he would feel better but he did not. Finally, he agreed to go to the dining room, he ate well, and told me on the way back to the apartment that he really enjoyed the meal very much.

He took a nap and when he awakened his legs were still hurting him. After calling the pharmacist, to see if the aspirin would conflict with the new medication, which the pharmacist said it would not, he started bleeding very profusely. I called Don, and he suggested calling to see if a doctor was on call. I had forgotten there is always a doctor on call for the weekends and holidays. I called security and told them in a very firm voice that I only wanted to speak with a doctor to see if I should take my husband to the hospital. Fortunately, Franklin Square Hospital is only about ten minutes away and practically a straight shot. The security officer, who was on duty, explained he would call the doctor on duty, and have her call me back. He did this and within five minutes the doctor called me. I explained the situation to her and she believed it was a urinary tract infection and he should have an antibiotic as soon as possible. She said she would call the prescription in to Sam's Club for us and I could pick it up as soon as possible. As it turned out, Sam's Club prescription department is closed on Sundays. The doctor called back for another suggestion for getting the prescription filled. We settled on Walgreen and I will pick it up in the morning. It was too bad that I didn't have a suggestion for picking up the prescription last night but we are all seniors, and not many of us like to go out driving late at night. I must give the doctor a lot of credit for her kindness toward me last night on the telephone. She is not our regular doctor, but her service was outstanding. I got the prescription this morning and there is a big improvement already. The bleeding appears to have stopped and Bob must feel much better judging from how he enjoyed his dinner.

Bob had two more bad falls, one about 5am and the other about 7am. He just can't remember not to get out of the bed in the middle of the night or early morning. He will fall every time. It is a wonder he can walk at all for as many times he has fallen on his knees. He goes down with such a loud thump that it is a wonder the people who live under us aren't awakened with a start. I am looking forward to a good night's sleep tonight and I hope I am not disappointed. It is amazing to me how Bob could fall so many times and not break any bones. Several times the Mobile X-Ray unit was dispatched to our apartment to see if Bob had any broken bones, after a fall, and we found there were no broken bones.

Wednesday, 14 June

What a day this has been. This afternoon, when I gave Bob his second antibiotic pill, for his intestinal tract infection, he spit it back into the glass of water, with the explanation that it had a bitter taste. I don't know what he expected. However, he then had to drink all of the water to get the pill back out. He had another bad night with his walking. It was really terrible and I still wonder if the medication makes it worse after it builds up through the day. It is now 1am and I hope we can get some sleep.

Saturday, 17 June

Bob was really mixed up mentally tonight. He said he was shaking and nervous as a kitten. I was making cole slaw in the kitchen, he was in the next room, watching the ball game. The Orioles were winning and he was very agitated. He said it was because I was grinding up the cabbage and the machine was making a noise, which wasn't very loud. He then came into the kitchen to watch and wait for me to finish so I could come into the other room and sit with him. Other than this, I think he had a pretty good day. He even wanted to go to the dining room for our dinner knowing that Jim was not going to be with us tonight. Usually, when Jim is busy elsewhere, Bob wants to get "carry-out" for our dinner, as we do every Monday when Jim goes to a meeting and dinner up at St. Joseph's Church where he does his Permanent Deacon work. I just wonder if Bob will feel better now that the infection is cleared up in his urinary tract. I certainly hope so.

Wednesday, 21 June

This is our 59th anniversary. Starting at 4am, Bob was up every half hour and wanting to know where everyone was, what happened to everyone and what was going on. He must have had some kind of dream that caused this confusion. Normally he is not so confused in the morning but today is the exception. He is in rare form. He is constantly calling and asking what is going on. We have to get started early today with shaving and his bath due to having the doctor's appointment. This change in Bob's routine may have been on his mind and caused him to be agitated. I expect lots of trouble with this change in his routine. The Stranger is still trying to enter Bob's mind and body earlier each day.

The extra twin bed, in my room, where Bob rests and watches TV, has dried out from being soaked last night. When he stays on his back, he remains dry as the bed does, but he is so restless that he rips the bed all apart. I am going to take his medication in now and I hope he will take a short nap.

Wednesday, 21 June — 1am

Bob received a very good report from his doctor today. He walked well and his balance was good. The doctor said how lucky he was to have done as well as he has, for having Parkinson's disease for fifteen years. He is taking the maximum amount of medication to help him. If he takes any more, he will have more of the shaking, like Michael Fox. It does build up through the day but this is what he needs. One lady, who lost her husband, said he went down hill and died in five years.

We watched some TV after dinner in the living room for awhile and then Bob started into the bedroom to continue watching and napping. He got part way when he fell and had to crawl the rest of the way. He got to the sunroom, where he decided to have some juice and his medication and could not get up into a chair. It took one hour to get him up into the wheelchair.

Later tonight, we went in to get ready for bed and he was in the bathroom, getting ready to use the water pick and down he went again on the tile floor. He finally asked for the security men to help get him up after we tried and tried for one hour without success to get him in the wheelchair. Boy was I glad. They came in and in one, two, three they had Bob up and in the wheelchair. I finished getting him ready for bed, where he is now, and tried to impress upon him not to get up, and out of bed, in the middle of the night as the same thing will happen and down he will go again.

Thursday, 22 June

Last night was unbelievable with seven hours of sleep for each of us. I guess we were both exhausted from all of the problems we had before going to bed. I will keep Bob in the wheelchair most of today and see how he is. I am also going to try and space his medication a little further apart to see if he keeps better control of his legs. I will try giving him two buffered aspirin in between his Parkinson's medication to see if that still helps him some. You almost have to be a detective to find the solution that works best for your loved one.

Today was good. Bob slept a lot, but that was fine. I did not awaken him to give him his medication. He had four doses rather than the normal six and in between I gave him the two buffered aspirin. I think he really made out much better. It may not work tomorrow or the next day but I will continue to play detective until we find the right amount. He did not have the cloud over his mind tonight and actually watched most of the ball game. I still used the wheelchair in the apartment for him to conserve his walking and will continue to use it until I am sure he doesn't need it.

Thursday, 06 July

Yesterday was just about the second worst day I have had as a "caregiver." Anything that could go wrong with Bob did go wrong. He fell near the bathroom door and was completely out of it as to how to get up. Every limb and muscle was solid and dead weight. I called the security people and two wonderful men came right up, and within minutes they had him up. They made sure he was not hurt and one, two, and three he was up and back in his wheel chair.

Later on in the day, he tried to make it to the bathroom, but failed to make it in time. He messed up everything possible himself, the toilet and the floor. All was cleaned up in a hurry and he was able to step over and into the Jacuzzi tub. He had a nice long bath, and he felt so much better. I am so glad we have a good tub. Sometimes he takes a shower but the tub bath seems to help his legs feel so much better.

We settled down for the rest of the day but it seemed like every time I turned around he was wet clear through. I don't know why the special briefs didn't work but they certainly didn't. Today he used six pairs of underwear plus the special briefs. I have said before that I am so glad we have a good washer and dryer and I don't have to run downstairs to wash clothes.

Well, we tried something different tonight. Instead of Bob riding in the wheelchair, from the second bedroom, through the sunroom and kitchen to his bathroom, I asked him if he wanted to try and push the wheelchair that he agreed to try. He started off with nice big steps and walked all the way to his bathroom. This made it so much easier for him to finish his teeth with the water pick. For years I have cleaned and brushed Bob's teeth by having him lie down on one of the twin beds, so I could reach all of his teeth, and then he would go into his bathroom and use the water pick. We got into this routine because his hands would shake so much it was difficult for him to hold the toothbrush. I got him already in the bathroom so that when he went into his bedroom he just had to climb in bed. Bob couldn't make it all of the way into his bedroom so he held on to the vanity and I turned the wheelchair around and he sat in it for the last 10-15 feet, which was very good for him. He can only stand for a short while but it was long enough for him to get ready for bed. I feel so encouraged to try this again. Even if it works some of the time it will be a great help for him and me. The chair, with him in it, is hard to push on the thick carpets. He had no trouble pushing the empty chair. I do hope he has another good night. He also pushed the wheelchair back from dinner tonight and did very well.

I still can't understand the strange feeling Bob has every night. He can't explain it very well, only to say that he feels so strange. He looks so bewildered when he discusses it also. As usual he doesn't want me to leave him to work on the computer or do anything in the other room. Finally, he will fall asleep and take a short nap and seems to feel much different when he awakens. Thank goodness he does feel better, as it is a bit scary when he speaks like the Stranger trying to control his life. It will happen one day, I just hope and pray I don't go first. I worry about him and how he would make out.

Saturday, 15 July

Everything is the same these days except Bob is losing the strength he had in his arms and legs. We still are able to manage okay but I don't know how long we can last. I do think some of these later days Bob has more control over his urination than he has had the last couple of weeks. The medication the doctor gave him for the pains in his legs does help and this is good. I still work the two buffered aspirin into his schedule of medications and it has made a big difference in his going to dinner and eating well. We still have the problem of him getting out of bed in the middle of the night and in most cases removing the special briefs that keep him dry in bed. They also help keep his bed dry. Many times he will deliberately urinate, with his briefs on, all over the floor.

Friday, 21 July

Thank goodness for the bells on the door. I had to put the bells on the handle to hear when he escapes into the hall. Once again Bob opened the door to the outside hall, and started to walk down the hall at five o'clock in the morning. He was very startled when I called to him and asked him where he was going. He had another dream and said he needed the police. I asked him "What did he need the police for?" He mumbled something that I could not understand. When I convinced him to return to bed, he requested a telephone. He kept asking me where the telephones were. Finally, I took hold of him gently and he awakened fully and said he had this awful dream. These dreams are so real to him. He is back in bed now and I hope he will sleep until eight o'clock in the morning. It is now six thirty and this is the third time he has gotten out of bed.

This evening has to be one of the worst, so far, for helping Bob get ready for bed and into bed. His legs will not hold him and I cannot understand why he is so helpless at night. It would seem, after having his medication all day, that he would be better in the evening and later at night. It took one hour and twenty minutes to get him from the bathroom into his bedroom and once I was able to get him into the wheelchair he could not get into bed.

He was dead weight with no control over the stiff arms and legs and in fact, the whole body had no movement at all. It was almost like he was paralyzed, which he was not. It is just the way Parkinson's affects the body. I know he can't help it but my arms and back and side really hurt from pulling and trying to help him.

I am not sure he will be able to stay dry tonight because of all the pulling and moving him from side to side, in the bed I am not sure his special briefs are on secure enough to really help him tonight. I hope he sleeps through the night and that will help him.

Monday, 24 July

Tonight was like one of those awful dreams with Bob asking me all kinds of questions about who my parents were, what was my maiden name etc.… He also thought there were two of us taking care of him. It is so strange how he gets like this every once in awhile.

I don't know what I can do about his urination on everything possible. He has ruined the kitchen chair by sitting on it when he was very wet. It caused all of the varnish to peel off. He got two of the beds wet, one where he sleeps at night and the other where he naps in the afternoon. And, then he tells me he was on my bed and got it wet. I am now doing three or sometimes four loads of wash every day. I have had to wash spreads, blankets, sheets and towels that he grabs in the bathroom to wipe up the floor when he misses the toilet. What a mess!!! I keep him in three sets of the "special briefs" now during the day. They just don't fit very well in the creases of the legs and cause the leakage which can make everything wet. Yet, he still tries very hard to be independent and do the correct things but he just can't help having these accidents. Tomorrow is another day and we will see what happens.

Thursday, 27 July

This has been one of those days you hope never to see happen. Bob had a very good night last night and got up this am and walked surprisingly well, with very long steps. Later on, in the morning, he had to go to the bathroom for his elimination. Well, he didn't make it in time. He had a mess everywhere, in his clothing, floor of the bathroom, toilet and then he even walked in the mess with his bare feet. I got a basin of water, with soap, and let him soak his feet, so I could clean them, and he would be able to walk into the walk-in shower, which is connected to the master bedroom.

I was surprised that he was able to walk after this upsetting episode, which he was very well. Finally, he had a nice shower, got cleaned up, and felt much better. Don, our son, came over later and I was telling him a little of what happened and I told him this was better to cope with than the constipation, which can still be a problem. As I told him, when all of the muscles are involved you can expect almost anything. Bob enjoyed his sandwich, which Don brought over, and we ended up having a very nice visit. Don is very thoughtful to come over, once a week, for a visit and to bring lunch. He and Barbe have really been terrific!

Monday, 07 August

The temperature of the apartment is very uncomfortable. Because Bob's illness makes him cold all of the time the thermostat is set high. He will be cold when it is in the nineties. I have windows open in places he isn't sleeping or watching television, but he wears long-sleeved shirts to keep warm and thankfully the apartment is heated/cooled in two regions so I can regulate it a little. Everyone who comes over understands but I tell them to dress accordingly. The summer is especially bad. I like it cool especially to sleep and he is always cold.

38

Friday, 29 September

It is hard to find time to write. Bob is getting worse.

Wednesday, 04 October

These two months have really rolled by quickly. Most things are about the same with Bob. He has had good and bad days with many accidents. Every once in a while he has had a good night, sleeping all night through and awakened in a dry bed and himself dry with the special briefs working fine. They work great when he can sleep on his back and there is no leakage this way.

He has started taking Goji juice, which is an all-herbal drink. It is good and tastes like strawberries. Jim thinks he is more alert since he started taking it about five weeks ago. I agreed with him up to tonight. He had one of those spells that he hasn't had for sometime now. When he awakened from a short nap he had a bad cloud over his mind. He just couldn't get it straight who I was and wanted to know where the other people were. He kept repeating the same questions to me try-ing to understand if I was a man, why I had on men's pants, and who my wife was. He wanted to make sure that he was a man and wore men's clothing. He said he had never tried to wear women's clothing. It was over an hour before he started to come around and act like he did know who he was and who I was. He seemed to have a clearer mind when he went to bed although he said it had not cleared completely. What a day! The Stranger will not give up. He is so persistent.

Tuesday, 10 October

Last night was one of those up and down nights that hap-pen frequently. Today started off pretty good and I thought it was really going to be a good one. Boy was I wrong! Bob had one of those episodes that he has not had for a long time. Since he had not had a complete elimination for a couple of days, he took his Milk of Magnesia last night. When he was headed for the bathroom today, he did not make it in time He messed all over the bathroom and the toilet and himself. What a mess! Never the less, we felt like at least he didn't have to worry about constipation today. All I can say again is "What a mess!" We started early tonight to do the cleaning of his teeth and to get him ready for bed. The brace on his one leg really works very well. It certainly helps his walking. I do hope he has a better night tonight than he did last night.

Tonight about eight o'clock Bob felt like the cloud was returning over his mind. However, he really wasn't too bad for it was an off night. I must call his doctor in the morning to see what he says about Bob's reaction to the Sinemet medication. Each time he takes the medication he has a reaction in about thirty minutes. He shakes all over, hands, legs and body. It is almost like he has taken too much but I know this can't be because I give his medication to him. Sometimes he takes it every two hours apart and sometimes he takes it two and one half hours apart. I do not see how he could be taking too much. This is five pills a day and sometimes six pills a day. We will see what the doctor says.

I am so glad I asked Bob's doctor if he thought braces on Bob's legs, at the knee area, would help to keep them from buckling under him and making him fall. His answer "Try them and see if they help." The doctor also suggested buying them at Wal-Mart where they are inexpensive to try. I did exactly that and they have worked very well so far. They are very tight and fit over the knees with good support above and below the knee. I think even though Bob does not like them on his legs, they do give him more confidence to walk.

Thursday, 12 October

Bob's doctor returned my telephone call and we spoke at length. He came to the conclusion that the Parkinson's disease was progressing but most of the trouble was the dementia, which usually happens to Parkinson's patients. He explained Bob had been very fortunate up to now that the dementia had not been a problem. He would like to see Bob in his office shortly and for me to call for an appointment. I am sure it will be very difficult to get Bob over to his office

Sunday, 05 November

What a day this has been. All of a sudden Bob's condition really changed. The cloud was over his mind, he didn't know where he was, didn't want to eat his dinner, legs so weak that he remarked he didn't know he was that sick, thought I was his brother Bill and wanted to know when his wife was coming back, other times his whole body, legs, arms everything were rigid and stiff as a board. It took one hour to get him ready for bed and another twenty minutes to get him in bed from the wheelchair and then he slipped down on the floor and had to crawl to the bed, which was about three steps away. Finally he could get up on the bed, on his stomach, and I lifted his stiff legs onto the bed. Then I rolled him over to get him situated so he would be comfortable when this spell wore off and I am sure it will wear off, at least this time.

What a shame when this happens after he has had some really good times recently. We both are exhausted.

I just went in to check Bob before I go to bed and found he is sleeping like a baby. He seemed so relaxed and I am hoping he will have a good night.

Sunday, 19 November

We have a small box sitting on a table, in my bedroom, which faces into the sunroom, that has a mirror in the top of the box, which also faces into the sunroom. Several times Bob had a bad hallucination that happened when he glanced over in the direction of the mirror, while lying on the twin bed resting, when he could see a Stranger's reflection in the mirror. He became very agitated, got off of the bed, and tried to fight the imaginary figure. One of these times he had a really bad fall and ended up with a bad bruise on his forehead. I could not reason with him that no one was in the apartment except us. I finally cut a piece of cardboard and covered the mirror by scotch-taping the cardboard over it. That problem was solved and he never had that particular hallucination again although he had many others.

Saturday, 09 December

Bob had a very good night last night but today he has just gotten weaker and weaker. He almost fell in the sunroom, right next to the glass doors in the center of the room. I was able to pull a chair behind him and he dropped into it. I then got the wheelchair and now he is watching André Rieu on tv. We have seen this program about five or six times but the music is so good and André Rieu is a real showman. This is what he likes and he is enjoying the program.

Bob has had many good nights since he started taking the Goji Juice once a day of only three ounces. It seems to make such a difference. His body changes very quickly and without any warning or reason as to why the changes happen so quickly. It doesn't make any sense to us but I think this must be the way Parkinson's disease works. Also, the medication has its drawbacks but if you must take it there is no alternative except to feel terrible with awful tremors, in his body and limbs. This is a terrible disease.

Sunday, 10 December

Bob was good the first part of last night. However, he had a terrible morning! Bob felt so bad that he really thought he was dying. Terrible me! I told him, very gently, that if he was dying he would just close his eyes and go to sleep and he would not know that he was dying. I also told him again that if he was tired of living with this disease to ask the Lord to take him home, when he says his prayers and if he wanted to stay with me a little longer to ask the Lord to help him with his Parkinson's disease. It seems to settle him somewhat when we talk like this.

I have decided not to go to the meeting luncheon on Tuesday. Bob seems to be having too many times when he is agitated these days. I wouldn't want him to have one of these and be by himself. It is just as well anyway since I have gotten out of going to these meetings and luncheons. I am busy enough here, where it is closer to home.

Wednesday, 10 January

Things have been going along about the same. Bob is slowly losing ground in his fight with Parkinson's disease. I must say last evening we were pleasantly surprised by the fact that for the first time in a very long time, probably months, he did not have the cloud over his mind. He was unable to fully explain what happens when he feels this cloud. He said he experiences something in his head that is uncomfortable and worries him. He said it does not feel like pain or pressure but he just could not explain what he feels at this time. Tonight was the usual situation that the cloud was there and he questioned where he was living now and who I was.

He was really out of it when he was using the urinal tonight and he had a complete elimination on the living room rug, which happens to be a fine oriental rug. It all cleaned up and I will check it in the morning. Then of course, it meant Bob had to have a shower because the mess was all over his back and legs. What a mess! However, I continue to pray for patience because I am sure he can't help it. I believe almost all control has left him. Once in awhile he seems to have some warning that he has to go to the bathroom and he will just about make it. Anyway, he is in bed now for the night and I do hope he can sleep through. He does not remember that he wears special briefs at night so he doesn't have to get up to go to the bathroom. Most of the time, when he gets up, he falls in the bathroom and that floor is tiled with no protection when he falls. Bob can usually take sixteen steps and down he goes. It must take this long for his blood pressure to drop down. He has been so lucky, when he falls, but I am sure his luck will not continue and he will end up with a broken hip or a bone somewhere.

These are some of the many problems that Bob has in his living with Parkinson's disease. My only hope, in keeping this journal, is that it will help someone realize these things seem to be normal for some one with this disease. You never have to panic when these situations happen. We are both eighty two years of age and I am sure that some of these problems could happen even if Bob did not have Parkinson's disease. Some of these accidents could very easily happen in the normal every day living with senior citizens. We have always been very grateful that Bob did not get this awful disease when he was thirty five years of age, like Michael J. Fox. This is a terrible cross to bear. Bob has had this disease for fifteen years and that is a long time. It is now 2am and I am off to bed and I do hope Bob continues to sleep.

Wednesday, 15 February

Things are not much better; in fact they are slowly getting much worse. The accidents continue in the bathroom and any other place that Bob happens to be. Once in a great while he has a brief warning and will try and make it to the bathroom. Usually, he sits crooked on the toilet so that there is a mess all over the toilet and generally urinates on the bathroom floor. He realizes this happens but says he cannot help it and I am sure he can't. Most of the time he will grab the clean towels and try to wipe up the floor, which I wish he wouldn't. He tries to be so helpful but he is not able to do most of what he was formerly able to help with when he had one of these accidents.

Bob continues to have these changes in his brain, like a cloud, in the evening. Tonight for the first time he was really nasty. He shouted "take our hands off of me!" when I had not touched him. I was close to him, as I usually am, when I take his arm to help him into the wheelchair. I do hope he doesn't become mean like so many people do when they are ill. The Stranger never misses an opportunity to try and control Bob's mind and body.

Bob slept much more during the daytime, and I wonder if his Parkinson's disease is progressing more rapidly now. He is taking Aricept once a day and I also wonder if he should have it twice a day, morning and evening. His mind is so clouded most evenings that he doesn't know who I am, when I leave or if I stay at night or where I sleep. He is so confused at this time of the day which he is not earlier in the day. I also wonder if the Carbadopa-Levadopa agrees with him now. I will have to question the doctor next month when he has an appointment. I remember Bob's doctor telling us that in many cases the Sinemet does not help the patient after he has been taking it for a long period of time.

Thursday, 22 February

If anyone reading this Journal has a loved one who is suffering from Parkinson's disease please keep in mind there are many changes in one who has this disease. All people suffering with this disease do not have the same symptoms. Many times when you think you have seen it all, or heard it all there is something different that can happen. I have been having very good luck in the evening when Bob has this cloud come over his mind. Last night my way of handling it didn't work

45

but for the most part it does. After dinner, when most of these episodes take place, about 6pm or so, I give Bob two regular coated aspirin, then in about a half hour I give him his regular scheduled medication. It is surprising how well this has worked to clear his mind and to also calm him. It has been a real challenge to try and work with the Stranger who is always trying to control Bob's mind and body.

Today was another one of those days that if something is going to go wrong it will go wrong. When Bob is in taking a morning nap, he is very restless and twists and turns a lot in the bed. As a result, many times he pushes his special briefs down so that they are no help at all, if he has an accident. He got up to go to the bathroom and had a trail through the bedroom, hall and into the bathroom. The mess was on his body, and legs etc....It has happened before but this was a pretty nasty job to clean up plus getting him in and out of the bathtub before his medication really kicks in to help him. Thank goodness we have a good washer and dryer in the apartment.

I have said repeatedly I pray for patience and the strength to continue giving care and help to Bob. I know he can't help it but there are a lot of things to get used to and accept that you must do without complaining. That is part of getting along and keeping peace within your own mind. I want no regrets with God or family when this is over for Bob.

Bob is asleep now and I will get ready to go to bed shortly. I am still wondering what tomorrow will bring in the way of surprises.

Thursday, 12 April

This was another terrible night. Bob started off, about nine o'clock again, very agitated that I would not move him back to the house we lived in when we were in Timonium. He took his fist and tried to hit me on the jaw, fortunately it missed.

(I will watch out for these temper-tantrums) He walked all around, half falling; his legs shaking like jelly for awhile. Then he went to the front door, walked down the hall, knocking on the doors of the other residents, who live here. His legs were still shaking so I put the wheel chair in back of him so he could sit down. He turned around and took hold of the two handles and began pushing the wheelchair down the hall. Finally, I was able to get him to sit in the wheelchair and I began pushing it to the front hall where the reception desk is located. He wanted a police officer so I knew I could call for a security officer there. He dragged his feet all the way making it very difficult to push the wheelchair. We eventually reached the lobby and there was a security officer there. After a few minutes he could tell what the problem was so he called for additional security officers. Four of them came to talk to Bob, take his blood pressure etc.... With his blood pressure over two hundred and seven, the security men thought it best to call for the ambulance and take him to the hospital, which they did. At the hospital, the doctor did all kinds of tests but found nothing wrong except he was so agitated. Finally, Bob began to calm down and they released him at 3am and we returned home.

What a blessing it was that I called our son, Don, to come in to help. He stayed at the hospital with us and was able to bring us back home to the apartment where we live. I will receive a call from the doctor's office to bring Bob down in the morning, which I will try to keep the appointment. What a night!!! Before we came home from the hospital, Bob was telling Don about the man in our apartment, whom he was fighting almost like he was fighting for his life. The man had on a green suit with a green hat, was a complete Stranger to him, and he turned and looked straight at me and said "He looked just like you." Naturally there was no one in the apartment except the Stranger who was trying and succeeding to control Bob's body.

47

This is the first time that I heard the expression "Sundowning." The doctor in the hospital emergency room explained to me that when the sun goes down the whole personality can change in Parkinson's patients. They can become combative and very strong from the rush of adrenaline. This was our first introduction to the Stranger although this Stranger had been trying to control Bob's mind and body for a long time. After I learned this information, I would ask Bob, when he was agitated, if the Stranger was in his body and he always answered yes but he couldn't do anything about it. Bob was helpless to the control of the Stranger.

Monday, 16 April

Bob is in bed for the night. He wanted to go to bed at eight o'clock and I dragged it out as long as I could. He would not take his two capsules, supplements, that I told him were for the pain he gets in his legs. He said he did not trust me and didn't know what I was trying to give him. So, I told him very quietly that he had to take his medication and when he was ready to let me know. Then we would get ready for bed. He fussed about this for awhile. Then I asked him if he was thirsty and said I would give him a nice cold drink of water when he asked me for his medication. I told him that nobody could force him to take medication that it was up to him when the pain in his legs got bad enough he might ask for it. Fortunately, he had his pain medication for his legs at dinner time. Finally, he asked me for the medication and said lets get it over with so we can get ready for bed. When I tucked him into bed, kissed him goodnight and told him I loved him. He said he could not understand why I played tricks on him. I just asked him to tell me goodnight, told him I would check him before I went to bed and left.

This was another night that was not so great!! Bob seems to develop a whole new personality about one half hour after he takes the Carbodopa-Levadopa medication. I am going to call his doctor in the morning as I believe he must have developed a reaction to this medication. He is nasty and even looks mean and formerly he never had a mean bone in his body. Parkinson's disease is really a terrible disease and has really changed my husband.

Wednesday, 18 April

This evening started off with Bob being very agitated but not loud or nasty with it. So, instead of giving him his medication, which I am sure he needed, I gave him the old stand-by—two aspirin. They took about one half hour to work but he then settled down. I did not give him the supplement, as I did not want to upset him with more pills or capsules, so he may not sleep too long. However, I think I would rather have him awaken me in the middle of the night and not be so loud and nasty, which is not the way he is normally.

He is in bed for the night now and I will check him out before I go to bed.

Talking Bob out of being upset and agitated really tires me out. But, at least tonight it worked. No, he did not have a good day. He seemed to have awakened on the wrong side of the bed and was restless most of the day. Tomorrow is another day.

I called his neurologist today and he called back when we were at dinner. He left a message that he will call again in the am.

Thursday, 19 April

The neurologist called back today and told me to continue the medication that Bob's personal doctor said to discontinue taking. The neurologist said to cut down on his Parkinson's medication, which I told him I had been doing, and he wants me to call him in about one week. This is like a guessing game with the doctors trying to prescribe the correct medication.

And how was he tonight? Well, he was almost as bad as the night he went to the hospital. He once again wanted to go back to his old house. He did not want to stay here any longer. He put one shoe on and one slipper on and said this was what he wanted to do. He put the remote control, for his blue power-lift chair, in one of his shoes, tried to pull the cable out of the chair and stuff the whole thing in the side pocket of the chair. When I told him he would ruin the chair and he would not be able to move it up and down, he said that was the way he wanted it.

He took the other shoe off and raised it over his head and tried to hit me with it. I told him "Don't you dare hit me with that shoe," which was a mistake. He said I will dare if I want to. He looked so angry that you would not believe it. Yes, sometimes he does scare me. He would not sit in his wheel chair but pushed it across the room. All the while I was trying to tell him to sit in the chair because his legs were so shaky that I thought he was going to fall. He wanted to push the chair down the hall again. I told him if he sat down in the chair I would take him anywhere he wanted to go.

We finally got Bob into his bedroom, he had to sit down in the wheelchair because he was so tired, but he would not let me help him get ready for bed. He just sat there and looked at me and asked me why I was playing these games with him. He also asked me if he didn't have the right to be afraid of me??? I kept telling him that he had no reason to be afraid of anyone. I was taking care of him and helping him to be more comfortable. Finally, after a half an hour he agreed to let me help him get ready for bed. I kept telling him what a good job Don had done in getting the bed back together, after the bottom rail was broken when he fell against it, and there it was waiting for him, all nice and fresh and clean. He finally got the picture. And, he is in bed for the night. I am worn out.

Oh, by the way, the neurologist said he is not having a reaction to the medication, that it was helping him, this was the dementia taking hold of him, which usually happens with people who have Parkinson's disease. He continued, that Bob has just been very fortunate up to now by retaining his clear mind. This is true because sometimes Bob could remember things that his brother and I could not recall quickly.

It is so strange that Bob can change so quickly. He ate a very good dinner and we came back and he took a short nap, in his chair. We were watching the news when all of a sudden he looked at me and started asking me "Why was I playing these games on him? What were these tricks that I was playing on him??" It scares me what might happen when I am asleep! I think Bob knew who I was last night, at the very end, when he was in bed for the night; he gave me a big hug. He didn't say anything then but the hug said a lot. He is so sad at times.

Oh, yes, Bob took off his protective briefs and threw them down the toilet. Fortunately, he didn't flush the toilet. I can't imagine what he will do next.

Friday, 20 April — 3am

Bob just awakened, at three thirty in the morning, and the first thing he said was "What are you doing here?" He finally awakened all the way and his mind was clearer. You can't imagine how sad it is. I know it is not Bob. It is a Stranger in the body of Bob. Help wouldn't do much good if he is fine and as soon as the help leaves he changes. I wonder if the worst thing I could do would be to bring in strangers to help take care of Bob. I think he would probably fight them like he was fighting for his life. He is unable to reason that they would be here to take care of him. I am not sure what the solution will be. Time will tell depending on how much he changes and when. He is back in bed now and I, too, will return to bed and see if we can both get some sleep.

Friday, 20 April

Today was a very good and normal day for Bob. He went with me to Wal-Mart, stayed in the car, while I picked up a few things. When we came home he sat on the bench, by the door, and watched me unload the car. I left his wheelchair in the hall, next to the first apartment door, with permission, which made it very quick and easy to get when we returned and came up to our apt. After I took the cart, with the groceries in it, to our apartment, I returned downstairs, where Bob was sitting on the bench in the sun. I joined him and we sat there for about a half hour or more and it was very relaxing and enjoyable. It actually was very restful.

Later we went to dinner and he ate pretty well and seemed to enjoy it. On the way home, riding in his wheelchair, he changed so quickly that Jim could not believe it. He said he was confused where we were and looked like he was very confused. The Stranger travels with us, at all times, and never misses an opportunity to try and control Bob through his mind and body. It may be another bad night. I just gave him the two aspirin and I am hopeful for a better night. I am still praying I make the right decision when the time comes that I will have to decide what to do next.

When I was making up the bed in Bob's bedroom this morning I noticed the telephone was off the base. I asked him if he wanted to make a call in the middle of the night and he remembered that he had been trying to get Jim on the telephone. Naturally, he did not have his number and goodness only knows whom he did reach on the other end of the line. I hope no one answered their telephone as it was three or four o'clock in the morning.

Tonight was another one of those terrible nights. Bob wanted the police and started down the hall whistling and calling people. I pulled the cord and got four security men who couldn't make much sense out of what Bob was saying. They called three paramedics who talked to him, and could not make any sense of what Bob was saying either. Finally, Bob said he wanted to talk to Jim so I called him and he came over. One thing the paramedics got Bob to take his emergency pill. He isn't asleep yet, but he has calmed down.

I pray for help to make the right decision, the next step. I hope I decide the right step to try and keep Bob satisfied and happy which he is not in this condition. The Stranger who tries to get into Bob's mind and body is a challenge and I am not sure who will be the winner to control Bob's mind and body.

Saturday, 21 April

We both had a good night's sleep last night. The Lorazepam, which the doctor gave me to use for Bob, in emergencies, worked to relax Bob enough that he was cooperative, in getting ready for bed, and without any more negative situations. He has been sleeping most of the day. He awakened once and I gave him his second dose of Sinemet, for his Parkinson's disease. He asked me if I had heard anything from our neighbors who may have been disturbed last night by his hollering and whistling down the hall for the police. I told him I had not but I was sure they would understand that he had a bad night.

The security men were so good with him, very kind and gentle. He says he does not want to go to the dining room tonight. I will see how he is later on in the day.

Don and Kathy just called from their car, as they drive to Villanova for their daughter Beth's dance recital. I am going to copy Don's last email message, to me, and place it below. I thought it was important to help me think this situation through and to make the right decision in caring for Bob.

53

"I am sorry this is happening to Dad and you. You will know when it's the right time to help Bob in a different way. This is the disease at work, you can't fight that, only delay it. You know, I think it was good Uncle Jim was involved, and maybe he should be involved some even though you think it makes him anxious, as he will be another voice to help you discern when it's time to take the next step with Dad. In my opinion I think you will need to hear from others around you with a little experience, so you can really look at the whole situation from all sides. Through prayer you will do the right thing, and you will know when it is time."

The Director of Social Services called this morning after receiving word from the Security office that Bob had trouble last night. She was very understanding and very easy to speak with. She has had a lot of experience with situations like this. She believes the next step will be moving Bob to the Assisted Living, on this campus, but across the road from the Independent Living. She will have the Social Worker get in touch with me next week. I also asked her to speak with Bob's brother Jim, who also lives here in the same community. Jim was here last night, when Bob was so agitated. I am sure he knows how the situation has developed and, by speaking with the Director, he may have a different perspective on the whole situation. I do not want to make any hasty decisions. So, now we will see how the rest of the day goes.

Saturday, 21 April — about midnight

We had an uneventful evening tonight. Bob was very quiet today and especially tonight. He was very cooperative before we got ready for dinner. I fixed the basin of soapy water for him to soak his hands and then his feet, which he was glad to do. I then cut his fingernails and toenails, cleaned him up with cream and cornstarch, mixed with some powder, shaved him, and he really looked good. You would never guess Bob had any problems. If all goes well tomorrow, I will trim his hair a little for him.

I believe the emergency medication (Lorazepam), must last him through most of the next day after taking it. I didn't think I would need to use it tonight until he started to get so tense and agitated. He continues to ask so many questions about the old house in Timonium. He still has that on his mind.

Bob picked over his food at dinner, which was unusually good, but he ate most of it slowly. I did notice he is cutting his food in very small portions, after I cut it for him, and chewing a long time before he swallows, which makes me wonder if he has trouble swallowing but I said nothing to him about the swallowing.

Tonight, I talked very quietly with Bob for forty-five minutes why he should take his last medication, (really the Lorazepam) to help him relax and to make him feel better, which it did. Finally, he asked me to give it to him. Within fifteen minutes I could see him relax and lean back in the chair. Then he asked if we could begin to get ready for bed, which we did. All went well with getting ready for bed and he is there now. I do not believe he is asleep as yet but I will check him in a few minutes to see if he is asleep.

Monday, 23 April

Last night as I was resting in bed half asleep I heard a noise that sounded like someone sleeping and breathing, in and out. I called out, softly, Bob is that you? I thought he had come into my bedroom and was sleeping in the other twin bed. I opened my eyes and there appeared a figure, at the foot of the other twin bed, which was so large that it went from the foot of the bed to the ceiling but leaning toward the bed sort of bent over the foot of the bed. Looking at it, I was not frightened, but I thought it was the spirit of Bob and that he had died. Please keep in mind; I was fully awake at this point.

I stayed there for a few minutes and then got out of bed to go into Bob's room to check him to see if he had died and there he was sleeping very soundly. I went back into my room and the figure was still there. My thinking at this time was it was a man and his clothing was off-white, but I could not see pants and a shirt. The clothing sort of went all together. The figure was still in the same position, leaning over the other twin bed. I got into bed, and said "Lord, if that is you, please help Bob. He is so miserable; take him into your care" and I continued to pray for a short while. Almost immediately when I finished praying I fell into a very deep sleep until 6am. I did not look at the clock when this happened but it was after twelve when I went to bed so I am sure it was late into the night. No, I am not going crazy! I know I was fully awake and not dreaming. I do not know what this means but I am sure it has some meaning for us.

Monday, 23 April — Later

I thought tonight was going well but then, close to nine, Bob had another spell where he looked at me and asked me what trick I was trying to pull on him. Where did his wife go?? He looked all around, with very shaky legs, finally fell and received a gash on his arm about ten inches long. (No blood, just scraped it) He sat in the chair for a few minutes and finally went to the door to find a policeman to find out what happened here.

Bob opened the door with me behind him, and we saw two neighbors in the hall. Bob tried to get them to help him but his speech was unclear. The one man was very kind to him and the woman went back into her apartment so she would not get involved. Finally, I asked him if he wanted me to call his brother, Jim, over and he agreed that he would come in and sit if I would call Jim, which I did. Before I called Jim, with the telephone in my hand, I asked him to take his last emergency medication before Jim came over. Finally he took it and put it in his mouth with some water. When Jim arrived and spoke with Bob it was all about Bob trying to figure out the situation that did not make a lot of sense to Jim. Before Jim left, Bob was very tired and weak and wanted to go to bed so we took him in to his room and by then he was cooperative. No doubt he is really weak but I do hope and pray he has a good night of sleep.

Tuesday, 24 April

Today was a very special day for me. I am so thankful that I did not have to miss the last Annual Meeting and Luncheon of the Woman's Eastern Shore Society. I enjoyed it very much and especially as I was honored, with flowers etc.., (I am the only member who has served as President three times.) and I was able to take some nice pictures that I would never have the opportunity again to take. I will also receive a video tape of the affair, which should be very nice. Many thanks again, to our son, Don, for staying with his dad because his doing so gave me a great deal of peace of mind that Bob would not worry with someone else in the apartment with him. I have always referred to this condition as "The Stranger trying to take control of Bob's mind and body" which was the best way for Bob to understand the changes in his mind and body.

Bob seemed to enjoy visiting with Don although he was very tired. He went to his bed, in his room, and slept for two and a half hours. I got carry-out for dinner, and he ate later. He did not eat all of his dinner because he was more interested in getting back to bed. He came out of his room after about a half hour and started in one of his temper-tantrums. About eight o'clock I was finally able to convince him to take his Lorazepam and he really calmed down and did not want to go to bed until 11pm. This medication causes the same symptoms as his Parkinson's disease and this is why the doctor said only to use it in an emergency. It is a sedative and it does calm Bob down enough to work with him. I needed something that works to calm him down when he gets very agitated. The doctors are calling it "Sundowning" as the doctor in the emergency room at St. Joseph's hospital called his behavior. There are many articles on the internet about this condition. I have always referred to this condition as "The Stranger trying to take control."

The social worker indicated to me that Bob would not qualify for the Assisted Living but he should at the Medical Center, which is like a Nursing Home. She did indicate that as long as he got his medication, I could probably take him home and return him to the Medical Center, either before or after dinner. We will see. As long as the sedative works, there isn't a problem here. I think they will probably use a sedative for him at the Medical Center. So, nothing would be different.

I am trying to get an appointment, with the social worker, next Wednesday to tour the Medical Center. Bob is settled for the night and I do hope and pray that he has a good night without the dreams and nightmares.

Wednesday, 25 April

I was getting Bob ready for bed and he fell down on the floor, although it was very slowly, he couldn't help himself at all, probably because he had the sedative at eight o'clock. He tried crawling from the second bedroom and got to the door, of the hall going to his bedroom, and he had a mental block about going around the corner. He tried and tried to finish crawling around the corner but he just couldn't make it. So, I pulled the cord and two of the nicest security men cane and picked him up, one two three, even though Bob was dead weight. They helped finish putting his pajamas on and lifted him into bed. Boy was Bob glad to be in bed, and I am very glad also. We started at nine o'clock to do all of this. It is now a little after 11pm. I guess I am just as tired as Bob---almost. I can see that we will have to get ready for bed before he takes that last pill. He is just lifeless and dead weight when he is like this. That sedative really works fast.

Thursday. 26 April

Bob just fell down again in the bathroom. He did not hurt himself this time but he is dead weight and I tried for an hour and we couldn't get him up. I pulled the cord again and two security people came. They were not the same people as last night but just as kind and gentle. Bob has a big red place on his forehead where he must have hurt himself last night. It is a shame to put him through this if it isn't really necessary.

I believe we have reached the time when I can no longer help Bob, especially when he falls. It probably isn't the right thing to keep him here when he may get better professional help at the Medical Center. The Stranger continues to make progress in controlling Bob's mind and body.

Thursday, April 26 — Night time

Bob was really agitated tonight. He yelled don't be so damn dumb! The pillow feels like Hell! I finally told Bob I did not like to hear him talk like that to me. I also told him if he continued to use that kind of language I was going in the other room. I told him that he had the Stranger in his body and he would have to get rid of him. He then asked me to sit by him and hold his hand, which I did. He was his old self after that. We talked about many things. He asked me what I was going to do when he died. This really broke me up and I told him that I would be ok. I would have Don and Kathy and Barbe and Paul and probably Jim who would look after me. He patted my arm and asked me why I was crying. I told him I hated to see him feeling so miserably and wished I could do more to help him. I also told him that over at the Medical Center they would have many people to help take care of him and help to keep him comfortable. He said that was good. I also asked him if he wanted to die and he said no. I asked him again to ask the Lord to help him with his Parkinson's disease when he said his prayers, which he agreed to do.

Bob tried really hard and was able, with my help, to get into the wheelchair. I then took him to his bedroom, stopping along the way to get his last pill, the sedative, which he took willingly. He got into bed without letting me change his pajamas etc... But I thought what difference does it make? I will change everything in the morning when he is fresh. I do not think he will get out of bed tonight, he is too tired. I am only going to give him the sedative when he is on his way to bed. I think it changes his personality among other things.

Bob did not eat much lunch but ate a very good dinner.

Friday, 27 April

I am not going to give Bob any more of the sedative because I think that is what the doctor meant when he said it will work against the Parkinson's disease. At one o'clock this morning, Bob was wide awake, sitting on the side of his bed, sliding half way down to the floor, when I found him. We worked for about an hour and I finally got him back on top of the bed. He had pulled all of the buttons off his pajama top and I don't know where two of them are. I guess they flew across the room somewhere.

This morning I just finished getting Bob off the floor in his bedroom, as I was trying to take off the wet protection briefs, which he didn't want the security men to see, and he slid down on the floor again. I was finally able to get him on his knees, where he could hold on to the bed, and I changed him. It wasn't easy but we managed. After he hung onto the bed, not the posts, he was able to stand for a brief moment and I pushed the wheelchair behind him. What a job! I am so proud of him because he really tries, when he is able. Now, he is played out and sitting at the table sound asleep, which I think he deserves as hard as he worked. We will now see what else happens today.

Friday, 27 April — about nine o'clock

We are both glad this day is almost over. Bob is in bed for the night, I hope, without the benefit of the sedative. He still went to bed thinking I was playing tricks on him. And, yet, earlier today he thanked me for helping him and doing so much for him. I told him tonight I didn't like hearing the Stranger that is in him speak and I wasn't going to listen to him. It wasn't long before he changed. When I told him I would be in later to check on him he said "He might be dead by then." However, he did tell me "goodnight" and that he loved me after I told him I loved him. That Stranger continues to try and control Bob's mind and body.

Saturday, 28 April

Please, if you are reading this Journal and a loved one has Parkinson's disease do keep in mind that sometimes these patients roam at night. I am now writing at 6am. I awakened and thought I heard a slight noise. I opened my eyes and turned my head around and there was Bob on the floor. We finally got him into the wheelchair and I got him back to his room and into his bed, where I hope he will stay now until about eight o'clock.

Saturday, 28 April — Later

Bob is in bed but I am sure he will be up before long. I have tried to impress on him the fact that he will only fall and for him to wait until I come in to check him, which I do frequently. This Stranger will not let him remember these directions.

I know Bob has said frequently that he does feel sorry for me having to care for him. He has said several times "Poor You" meaning that he worries what will happen to me. I can tell him that I don't want to listen to the Stranger that is in him, when he has what I call his temper tantrums. This Stranger is awful when he makes Bob change so quickly.

He didn't eat but a small cup of soup for lunch. He ate very little of his dinner tonight. I did get him to eat some ice cream after dinner. Just before I got him into bed he ate an orange, cut up small, and an apple, cut up small. He is terribly weak but he did manage to help me a little, when I got him into the wheelchair and then into bed. When he can, Bob tries so hard to help himself, even to the point of raising his blood pressure dangerously high. He is usually soaking wet and I am also. It is a real struggle most of the time but we do have some successes.

Bob was somewhat confused tonight but he didn't get violent, which was a big help. I think the sedative makes him sleepy and more confused. I did not use it tonight. I am sure Bob can feel the change that comes over him when he takes the different medicines. He has always had a bad reaction when new medicines are introduced into his system. I feel terrible when I have to give these medications to him so he can calm down. I am sure he has a different feeling inside that I cannot help him to eliminate.

Sunday, 29 April

Early this morning, about 4:15am, I felt a slight tap on my right shoulder, which awakened me for I was not sleeping soundly. This right shoulder would be on the side next to the spare twin bed. I thought, in my sleepy state, that Bob had come into the room and climbed onto the other twin bed. This did not happen. When I opened my eyes I saw another vision, which was huge. The figure had his back to the room, this time. I could see his leg, which seemed to touch the twin bed and going up to the ceiling I saw his body and his shoulders, arms and head. Against the wall, away from the room was a small light. I believe there was a light the last time I saw this figure, when he was facing into the room. I was fully awake this time as I was the last time.

For some unknown reason, I clearly had the impression the figure was a male. I watched for a few minutes, prayed for help for Bob, got up and went into the bathroom, came back and got into bed and the figure was still there. I said some more prayers, begging for help for Bob, and then decided to go into Bob's room to check on him. I didn't know if Bob had died and this was his Spirit or not. I slipped into Bob's room and he was sleeping soundly so I went back into my room, got back into bad and the figure was still there. I did look at the clock again and it was getting close to five eighteen. I prayed some more and watched the figure slowly disappear. I rolled over and went immediately to sleep and I believe it was a very sound sleep.

I do not know what this might mean but I am sure it means something to this family. Bob is very weak and eating very little. However, I have never thought he was in the immediate state of slipping away and returning to his maker. Only time will determine what this means. Bob goes to his doctor tomorrow and maybe we will get some answers from him as to what condition Bob is in now. I know from my view but that is not a professional view. He is still sleeping a lot but doesn't get any strength from it. In fact, he is probably getting weaker from the lack of exercise, which he is unable to do now.

Bob fell down only once this morning. I was finally able to get him over on his stomach so he could crawl over to his bed, which was very close, and hold on to the bed and try to stand. He was able to do this, I slipped the wheelchair behind him and he was able to sit on it. I know he really needs more help now than I can give him. His arms hurt him from pulling and falling and a combination of reasons. I am also unable to get him into the tub to soak; he won't have the benefit of that. I did try the heating pad last night but it was uncomfortable for him so that didn't work either. I will rub his legs today with lotion and maybe that will help him.

Tuesday, 01 May

Today was pretty good for Bob even though he did sleep a lot. He awakened and came in for juice and medication (he never eats breakfast early) and went back to bed for two hours. I took about six small cups of soup that were frozen and put them into the blender, doctored them up a little with some seasonings and Bob was able to drink his lunch with some crackers. He seemed to really enjoy this for a meal. Since he hasn't been eating well I will continue to do this with his veggies etc....I also had some of the soup this way and thought it was delicious. Then after lunch, he went back to bed and slept for two more hours.

Dinner tonight was great! Bob ate the regular portion of spinach and mashed potatoes and two thin slices of cheese-cake with a tall glass of milk. Really a lot for him! I froze the chicken for sandwiches later on. He did not want any meat today nor did I.

This was a bad evening and night for Bob as he was very agitated and I couldn't get him settled down so I gave him one half of the first medication, the Lorazepam, and it didn't help him at all. In fact, it made him completely helpless. He went down when I was trying to get him from his chair into the wheelchair to get ready for bed. I tried for thirty minutes to get him back up but was unable to. I am now wearing one of the heat patches on my back and taking Aleve. I am not sure how I hurt it but I can guess so I am trying to be as careful as possible. I had to get the security men to help get him up. It took three of them and they got him into the wheelchair. He told them he did not want to go to bed, which was fine because he was too upset to sleep.

Bob then wanted me to call his brother, Jim, over, which I did once the security men had left. Jim came over and visited for a short while. Bob was telling him he needed a ride home from the Washington Stadium and to bring his car. Jim asked him how he got over there and he said Jane took him over there but left him. He was really played out and said he wanted to go to bed so we took him into his bedroom and boy what a time to get him into bed. I was so glad Jim was here but at the same time I was afraid he was going to hurt himself. After all, he has had two major surgeries. He said he did not hurt himself but Bob is really dead weight. I can only hope that he will sleep through the night now. Tomorrow is the day for the Tour of the Medical Center. Jim is really pushing for Bob to go over there as he knows I have done my best but it isn't enough now.

Thursday, 03 May

Tonight Bob ate very little for his dinner. He seemed alert and acted like he was no longer under the spell of the Valium, which had to be used last night. On the way home from the dining room there were changes in Bob literally as we walked along. Bob seemed to be agitated about something so I asked Jim to slow down a bit pushing the wheelchair. Jim is used to walking fast and it does not agree with Bob after he has eaten his dinner. Sometimes Jim knocks the wall or cuts a corner too short and Bob does not seem to tolerate this very well.

When we were sitting in the reception room, after dinner, Jim noticed the change in the way Bob looked with his mouth and eyes. He looked angry as I looked at him and I thought there was going to be trouble tonight which Jim and I both agreed.

As soon as Bob and I returned to the apartment at five forty-five, I gave Bob a whole pill of Valium, which I felt would help him sleep through the night. Well, in less than ten minutes he really became a madman. He grabbed my arm and started to hit me again, and succeeded. I then told him I wasn't going to get near him anymore for this Stranger to act up again tonight. He walked into my bedroom, with me a safe distance behind him, with his legs shaking; he got over to one of the twin beds, and could barely sit on the bed. I asked him to get all the way on the bed, so he wouldn't fall off, and he said "Shut up woman." I have never heard Bob use this expression in almost sixty years of marriage.

Eventually, he slid off of the bed, grabbed one of the tins holding thread, dumped the thread on the floor and banged on the bed for one half hour with the empty tin. He tore all of the covers off of one of the twin beds and tried to reach over and do the same thing to the other bed, which he did only partially. He threw pillows and was a real terror. The strength he had in his arms and hands was unbelievable. This must have been due to the adrenaline, as the doctor in the hospital had told us was the reason for this unusual strength that Bob had when he was agitated. The Stranger was in his glory tonight.

I kept asking him if he wanted help and he started to yell. I tried in between his yelling to get him to settle back on the bed where he would be safe from hurting himself, which he would not do. Eventually, he asked me to help him. I told him I would if he put his hands behind his head so he could not grab me again. He said he would not hurt me again and he wanted to get up. He said, "I give up. Please help me." I did for about fifteen minutes, after I hugged him and tried to relax him, but we just couldn't get him up. I am sure the Valium had kicked in by then and he was starting to settle down. This whole episode took about one hour and a half. I asked him if he wanted me to call the security people in to help us get him up and he agreed, which I did, and they were wonderful with him. One man picked him up by himself and the other lady helped with the wheelchair. They then took Bob into his bedroom and one, two, three had him in bed, where I hope he will stay for the night. He does not like the security people to come in to help him so I kept telling him that I would have to call them back if he got out of bed, which he said he would not do. I thought he would be asleep by now but I was just in there and he was not asleep yet. I think he was exhausted but too agitated to sleep. I believe the Stranger has won and is now in control of Bob's body and mind.

I called Jim to come over and help but I was sure he was still in the dining area visiting with some of his friends so I am sending him one of these updates so he can see what he missed, (haha) It is a wonder I have any humor left in me but I keep telling myself this is not Bob but a Stranger who entered his body. He leaves when he is sleeping at night and returns the next evening after the sun goes down. The doctor is sure he can control Bob but it will take some trial and error with medication. My prayers are that Bob can get the help he needs from the professionals quickly so he will not be too unhappy. Tomorrow is moving day for him. He said tonight, when he was agitated, that he will not go. I am glad Don is coming over. I think Bob may be better in the morning. We will see how things go. I am going in now to mark his clothing that he will take over to the Medical Center tomorrow. I know this will be one of the worst days of my life. I always said I would never take Bob to the Medical Center, but I know now he really needs professional help and I cannot do any more for him except get him the best professional help possible.

Oops, too late. I just heard a noise and went in to check on Bob and he was out of bed, sitting halfway on the chair in his room. I tried to get him back in bed but he fell down.

67

So, I asked Bob if he wanted the security people to help him again and he said I guess we have to have them. I agreed and two of the nicest men returned. One, two, and three he was back in bed. If it happens again, that he gets out of bed, the security people will call the doctor on call to see if Bob can take the other Valium. This is probably why the doctor did not give him one pill, as I requested, but two of the pills. I will try again to get his clothes marked now.

I have slipped in several times to check on Bob and he seems to be sleeping soundly. I do hope it continues for the entire night.

The Nursing Home Experience

Friday, 04 May — Moving Day for Bob

I have just returned from dinner with Jim. I thought this morning went very well. However, as good as the morning was, the opposite was true this afternoon and evening. Bob started much earlier today. When I went back to see Bob after lunch, he was with Jim and just acting terrible. The nurse put a tracking device on him that sounded a loud noise every time he broke the connection and tried to get out of his wheelchair. He finally got both medications about two forty-five. I can only hope the medication will make a difference. I went in to say good bye and he told me to get out and tried to kick me. This was while a doctor's assistant was putting a thermometer in his mouth. He was so upset that he pulled the cord around her neck that was holding the stethoscope. I hope they can handle him.

The chest x-ray yesterday showed Bob has the beginning of pneumonia, that they will treat. And, by the way, the aide said Bob did eat a good lunch.

Friday, 04 May — 7pm

Jim and I just returned from a visit with Bob. He was sedated but so nice and loving. I truly believe he will sleep through the night now. The nurses are so good to him. One of them had him in the hall near her office. She said she was moving him in her office and would take him to his room soon. She had given him the first dose of medication for the pneumonia.

If he were still home I would not have known he had pneumonia. I feel better after this visit. I told him I would see him tomorrow, Saturday early. Poor Jim is so worried.

Saturday, 05 May

Bob was very upset this morning, so the nurses gave him a medication that somewhat calmed him down. They called me before I got over there to tell me that he had fallen after he got out of his wheelchair and had a nasty cut on the bridge of his nose.

I got over to the Medical Center about 10:40 and was able to help him eat his brunch, which was an omelet, two slices of bacon, glass of milk, cup of applesauce, and a cup of vanilla ice cream and seemed to enjoy it. Later the nurse told me he had eaten a bowl of cereal, danish and juice earlier.

The nurse gave him his Sinemet and in ten minutes he was asleep for two hours in a type of lounge chair on wheels. Jim came over and we had a nice visit.

The nurses awakened Bob to change his brief and clean him up. Two nurses took him into his own room to do this. Jim and I waited where we were sitting in the hall. In a few minutes we could hear noise coming from his room and two other nurses, or aides, went in to help get control. Bob was fighting all of them, trying to kick, bite or do what he could to protect himself, as he told me later. He didn't know what they were going to do to him. I heard the nurse tell him but he may not have understood what she said. After much talking to him, we thought he understood that he had to let them help him so he would get better. But that was not to be the case because the Stranger, who is always trying to take control of Bob's mind and body, will not let him remember.

Friends stopped over to see Bob and me and they were carrying a very large bunch of roses and beautiful flowers. They were surprised to see how bad Bob looked and how he had started to lose so much weight. Jim and I had a nice visit with them although it was a short visit. Bob went back to sleep and continued to sleep while we talked. Jim and I left after a short while to return to Independent Living area for our dinner and I told Bob I would return at 7pm.

It is now six o'clock and I received another call from the Medical Center that Bob was fighting everyone, kicking, hitting, and biting, whatever it would take to free himself from their care. They could not get him to take any medication so they called the doctor, who was on call, and he ordered medication by needle to see if that would calm Bob down some. The nurse, who called me, was preparing me that I might see bruises on Bob, especially on his neck, where he tried to pull his clothes off. If this continues, they may not keep him but send him to Sheppard Pratt Hospital where they may have more experience with this type of behavior. I am leaving now to visit with him. Goodness only knows what I will find.

Sunday, 06 May

Bob did sleep through the night. The sedation is working and he had it twice today. Things are going OK for him now. He didn't eat much but that is fine. He is not doing anything but sleeping. He did have oatmeal, Danish, and orange juice this morning, which is good. I did get a little ice cream in tonight that had a crushed Sinemet (Parkinson's disease medication) in it. They are still using the needle, in Bob's hand, for the other medication. Don was in and had a nice long visit with his dad as well as Jim, Bob's brother. It is so sad to see Bob just lying there sleeping from the medication that sedates him. I know this is better than seeing him trying to get up and fall again. He is so frustrated with everything new, strange, and with strangers, nurses and aides, taking care of him. From time to time I have wiped tears from his eyes. His legs will not support him now. He looked clean, dressed, and well cared for again today. He also smelled good. The only thing I have requested for the nurses and aides is to keep him clean and comfortable and they are doing this. He has always been such a good man and it really hurts so badly to see him in this condition. I have always maintained that I would do anything to keep him home and not have to send him to the Medical Center. When he developed the Stranger in his body I could no longer cope with this change in him. The violent behavior was so bad I just couldn't handle him for which I am so sorry. I pray every chance I get that the Lord will continue to be kind and understanding with Bob and not have him continue to suffer so much.

Monday, 07 May

The nurses told me the doctor had changed one of his medications to help him. Bob really gave them a bad time this morning. He was very restless today, when I was there, but not as bad as earlier. He did sleep a little while I was there. Jim was trying to get him to eat some when I got over there today. I did his laundry while I was there today and that was nice.

The nurse also told me that Bob was in the final stage of Parkinson's disease and there is no way to tell how long he can tolerate this as he is so strong, and she has seen many cases of Parkinson's patients. I told her that the Neurologist has been telling me that if Bob didn't have the bad balance problem, he would be in early Parkinson's. I told her I guess the Neurologist thought that was what I wanted to hear. He was so wrong!

The nurse, who is not an RN but studying and will take her Board exams next year, also looked me straight in the eye and said they couldn't understand how I could take care of Bob this long. I told her it was determination to try and help him. I told her also, I thought they were keeping him nice and clean and he smelled so good. She said he better smell good and be clean or else they would know why not. The whole place is so clean without the usual smells you find in a nursing home.

The nurse also said they believed they can get him to level out to a different stage where he might be a little more relaxed and accept things better. She did not believe the doctor called in for consultation would change anything to speak of. She said Bob was a classic case of Parkinson's disease in the final stages.

Monday, 07 May — Evening

Tonight when I went over to see Bob, the aides had him all tucked into his bed. He was sleeping and looked peaceful. He was not fighting the world or himself. I brought his clean clothes home so I could press them a bit and make them more like what Bob is used to wearing. I will continue to do this. It is too difficult to find washing machines and dryers that are not in use at the Medical Center so I will begin to bring his laundry home to wash each evening when I return home.

Tuesday, 08 May

Bob was about the same today. He ate next to nothing and appears to me to be having trouble swallowing. They have done all kinds of blood work, checking for urinary tract infection with urinalysis, checking red and white corpuscles and found nothing wrong. So far, they are still saying Bob is in the "end stage of Parkinson's disease." Bob was put back into his bed for a nap when I was over there earlier. I had to leave to do paper work, signed about a hundred papers, in the Admissions Office, which was not taken care of last Friday.

I was trying to feed Bob but he ate next to nothing although I could hear his stomach making noises like he was hungry. He has either given up on eating or unable to swallow. I do not like the sounds I heard, in his throat, when he was lying down in bed. He is very weak but gets a little energy now and then and still tries to get up. He is fighting himself so hard. I only wish he could know what good care he is getting, but he can't. It is almost impossible to understand his speech now. I will go back shortly and see what is happening. I can understand when Bob says yes or no and once in awhile a few words and that is all. I tell him he has his mother's soft and low voice which I am unable to hear. This is equally difficult for both of us.

Tuesday, 08 May — Later

Bob was in bed, dressed for the night, clean and nice smelling. He kept his eyes wide open for a long time. I thought at first he was sleeping and I just turned on the bathroom light and I think he heard a noise. He made no attempt to speak but looked straight at me for a long time and held both of my hands in both of his hands. I put some water on his lips and he seemed to want that although he did not want a drink. I told him I would be back tomorrow and he looked like he would sleep. I just sat with him and cried and cried and I am hoping he couldn't tell. Every once in a while he would squeeze my hand. I wondered if he wanted me to help him up but I couldn't tell for sure so I just told him his legs wouldn't hold him until he got stronger and that the pneumonia had made him so weak. It is so sad! I wish he knew what good care he is getting.

Thursday, 10 May

Today was much the same as yesterday except that Bob appears to be having more difficulty in swallowing. It was so sad tonight when I was trying to give him some ice cream, it just lay in his mouth. His eyes were both open and he looked like he was just staring at me. I am not sure if he is able to focus his eyes now. Every once in awhile he seems to have tears in his eyes. Gently I wipe them away but it is so difficult to watch. He is being cared for so well that I could not complain about this at all. The aide has so much compassion. When she was telling me how she nursed him today that she also shaved him and even brushed his teeth. I have always been so proud of his teeth and the care that he always gave them. It also helped that he never smoked. I pray all day long for the Lord to hear our prayers and come to his aid now. He is so helpless that this is the only help he really needs.

Sunday, 13 May

Bob is getting a little better now; at least it seems the pneumonia must be getting better, because they are cutting back on his medication some. He is more alert and has his eyes open all of the way. His back hurt him last night and I couldn't understand why it still hurt him after the aides got him into bed. As it turned out, the aides in the morning had left the back pack in back of him in the chair all day long. This is like a pillow, only it has two steel pieces that are up and down in it to assist this machine that lifts him from his bed into the chair or from the chair into his bed. I am anxious to see if he had any redness or places where the steel pieces had cut into his back. He was trying to ask me to remove this thing, for want of a better name for it, but I could not understand him. I thought his back was tired, from sitting in the chair all day, and I was gently rubbing his back. I felt just awful because I did not understand him. His speech was a little better but not back to normal. I will be sure and check it every day from this day forward. Other than this mishap, he is getting excellent care and I have no complaints at all. He is clean and smells very good. He even had a very good shave today. I will stop over later to check on him. It is so good that the Medical Center, where Bob is now, is so close that I can walk back and forth to see him.

Tuesday, 15 May

Tonight was awful for Bob. He fought like a tiger to get out of bed for one hour and a half. He grabbed the nurse's arm and pulled and pulled trying to get up. He spit his medication out and I am not sure he got enough to help him. The nurse also tried to get him to drink a little water that he spit out. The nurse said he really needed some water. They are afraid he will become dehydrated without more water. He did get both feet out onto the floor several times and I put them back on his bed. He cursed and took a swing at the nurse several times. I sat in the darkened room just watching him to make sure he was unable to get out of bed. He would try and try to pull up, rest a few minutes and then try hard again. Finally, he was able to get onto his side and it appeared he was ready to give up and fall asleep. I guess he was really exhausted. The Stranger never gives up and continues to try and take over Bob's mind and body. The nurse said she might have to give him the medication by needle, which they do by putting the needle, with medication, into the vein in the top of his hand. I do hope he sleeps tonight.

Thursday, 17 May

Bob was in a good mood when I went back today after walking Don to his car earlier. About 3pm he ate two small bowls of lemon pudding for me. Snacks are given out from 2-3pm. Then at dinner he didn't eat much at all. In fact, tonight after Bob was in bed the nurse, not an aide, brought his plate of food down and got him to eat a small amount of food,

76

not much, but a little. She really tried hard to get him to eat. The same nurse got him ready and in bed tonight and she did such a nice job.

Bob looked so good after his shower today. I told him I wished he felt as good as he looked. He is still having trouble swallowing and this could be the reason he does not eat well. Also, he doesn't get any exercise so he probably doesn't have any appetite. He is so unhappy and all he talks about is, "I want to come home." When he asks me, "How Could You Do This To Me?," it really breaks me up. I wish he could be back home but I know what will happen as soon as the medication wears off. It is just impossible when he needs professional help; you have to accept the fact that the professionals can help him more than I could. They are giving him such good care that I have no complaints except I wish I could have helped him more. I was unaware of "sundowning" and did not know what it was until I researched it on the internet. I told him regularly "It was a Stranger in his body" that I could not cope with. I do hope he sleeps tonight because then he is not fighting himself or the world.

Friday, 18 May

Bob is a little better today. He slept some while I was there, ate good at the Brunch time, which is ten to twelve, ate nothing at 3pm snack time, while I was there, ate about fifty percent of his dinner tonight. He was wide awake when Jim was there and when Jim told him he was leaving Bob asked him to come back. Jim told him he had to do some writing for tomorrow and Bob said okay. Later when I told him I was leaving to eat and I would be back later, after he ate his dinner, he asked me not to be long. He also told me he would try and eat his dinner, which he did.

Bob needed no medication tonight and he was sleeping in his bed and looked so peaceful that I did not awaken him. I did sit with him, in the dark, for awhile and then brought his laundry home. I felt like he would sleep through the night. He looked so clean and comfortable.

Saturday, 19 May

Things were about the same with Bob today and this evening. I think he was more alert in the late afternoon. After Jim left he ate a small cup of applesauce, small box of milk, one half of his tuna fish, that was mixed up for him, no bread, and the inside of a chocolate éclair. He does like the custard filling.

When I went back tonight, it was about one hour and the aide came in to get him ready for bed. She brought the lift to help lift Bob into bed. I explained again and again, to him, how she would not hurt him and the purpose of the lift but it still seems to upset him. His eyes are very large and he looks so frightened. The nurses are giving him his blood pressure medication, to raise his blood pressure, but they did not give him the sedative tonight. He was very sleepy so they may have given it to him earlier. I do wish he could understand what good care he is receiving. He looks so good. I keep telling him that I wish he felt as good as he looks. He looked so peaceful after the aide finished washing him and got him into his bed.

Sunday, 20 May

Bob was about the same today and tonight. He ate very little but did drink a small glass of water for me today. It isn't much but it was something. He had several occasions where he had his eyes closed and a big smile came across his face. I guess he was seeing the angels. He made out well when the aide got him ready for bed. He even tried to help her take off his pullover, which was nice. When the aide had him still on the lift, she was changing the brief, and going to wash him, he was all in position to go to the bathroom, and I was thinking this, when, yes, he went all over the floor. The aide quickly slipped a brief under him, and on the floor. He seemed pleased with himself. No one said anything. When the aide left, I told him I bet he would be more comfortable and he agreed. Bob had been very concerned that he was going to have an accident in his pants, when Jim was visiting with him today. I had to keep reassuring him that he was well protected with the "overnight briefs" that he wore when he was home. He finally accepted this but he still seemed uneasy. He probably held himself through the afternoon, until tonight and without any exercise, I guess this was possible. He is so clean and particular that it is hard for him to accept this way of life. I can see no other way for him to be clean and comfortable, without being wet all of the time. The aides do seem to have a regular schedule for changing him.

For the first time, tonight, I saw what appeared to be a boil or abscess on the left side of Bob's back, about near the top one third of his back. It is about the size of a dime with a hard center, which looked like it could contain pus. The night nurse is calling in the professional nurse practitioner in the morning to look at it. I looked boils up on the internet and they say most are cause by bacteria infection. As it turned out this happened to be a mole and nothing else. When the aides were helping Bob to get onto his bed, they were holding him so that part of the skin was slightly pulled to the side, from the belt which is used on the lift, and this gave the appearance of a problem mole. I rechecked Bob's back and there were not any boils anywhere.

Tuesday, 22 May

Things were about the same today, with Bob. He slept a lot today but he did eat his early breakfast and ate about half of his supper tonight. The dietician was in today and the oatmeal that Bob eats in the morning is fortified and the mashed potatoes that he eats are fortified. This may help him some. The dietician was trying to get some idea of more foods that Bob might like. Naturally, they are trying to get him to eat more. He has lost almost three more pounds.

Tonight when I went back over, after supper, Bob was in bed sound asleep. I kissed him goodnight twice but he did not wake up. I sat with him for about a half hour and then brought this clothes home to wash. I hope and pray that he has a good night.

Friday, 25 May

Today was about the same with Bob. Jim was over today to visit with Bob and as soon as he left Bob opened his eyes wide. I really hated to leave him, at this time, because he had slept most of the time I was there. He asked me not to leave but I tried to make him understand it was his dinner time and also mine. I also told him I would be back after I ate my dinner and he finally said ok. I doubt if he will eat much dinner as he ate everything that was on his plate, including soup and milk, at the brunch hour. I did get him to drink a small glass of water, which was mighty good for him.

Boy, am I glad I went back over this evening. We were having a nice visit, as usual when he hasn't gone to bed; I washed his hands, face, and took his socks and shoes off and washed his feet thoroughly. He was saying something that I could not understand and he started to call for Aunt Marg. I asked him if he saw her, thinking he might have drifted off to sleep for a few seconds, but he said no. He called for her several more times but I could not understand why he said he was calling for her. He told me that he knew who I was and that I was there with him.

In a little while the aide came in with the lift to get him ready for bed. I explained to Bob what was going to happen because I have always felt the lift frightened him. He was very cooperative in helping the aide take off his clothes. She got him on the lift and was adjusting everything, which only takes a few minutes, and had him ready to put him on the bed when she noticed his legs were bent and his feet were not in place. She went to help him place his feet on the pads, and she noticed something was wrong. Bob had gone to the bathroom everywhere. I told the aide he had passed out. I really thought this time he was gone. The aide was afraid he was going to choke to death. He just hung on the lift machine, limp.

He was dead weight and his color was drained from his face and he started to turn purple. The aide needed help to get him off of the machine onto the bed. She screamed for help repeatedly. Four aides came running in to help her. Two or three RN's came in to help and they called for the ambulance with two paramedics all rushing in to help within minutes. Bob seemed to me to be unconscious longer than when this happened before. The aides finally got him onto the bed and he was like a sack of flour. They straightened him out and raised his head onto a pillow.

The paramedics asked me if I wanted them to take him to the hospital. I said no that neither one of us wanted a hospital trip in a situation like this. So, the paramedics took his blood pressure, which I forgot, but it was unusually low. By this time, Bob was coming out of it very slowly and began to gasp for air. After a few minutes he stopped gasping for air, the purple color started to leave his face and he began to return to his natural color. He appeared to be on the road to recovery.

Everyone finally left and one nurse and the aide finished getting Bob ready for bed and Bob appeared peaceful, clean and comfortable. I sat with him for awhile and he finally rolled over and went to sleep. The nurse brought in the oxygen machine and Bob was given some aid for his breathing.

I am glad I was there. When a representative from the Medical Center calls about a problem that happens in the Medical Center, it is after the fact and you never hear the full story. He had wonderful attention and it was immediate. I can find no fault. The muscles in his legs are not able to support him any more. He cannot stand on the lift or walk.

One good thing did come out of this happening tonight. The aides will not use the lift machine anymore to put Bob in bed. They will use two aides or a nurse and an aide. This I was promised and I will make sure the machine is never used again on him. I am looking forward to the committee meeting next Tuesday. This meeting will be a question and answers meeting with all of the people who help take care of Bob. I am writing down some questions to ask.

This is the response from our son, Don, who has been very supportive and thoughtful.

"I am sorry you both had to go through this but it sounds like they really took good care of Dad. He may have more "pass out" episodes coming; I know you are prepared for that. God is watching him...Love Don"

I am sending a copy of this email to Jim because it was very upsetting and will save a lot of talk about it later; after all, I also know he is interested in what happens to his brother. I am including his response to this email, which I thought was very meaningful. I have always appreciated his support.

"Jane, I got up about 6:30am and on a whim I checked my internet messages. Your message about Bob glued me to the screen. Until the end of the message I was terribly anxious of what the outcome was going to be. It was a relief to hear that medical assistance was so prompt and in numbers. The "happy" ending was that Bob returned to some kind of normalcy and finally went to sleep. It was fortunate that you were there and gave support to Bob and direction to the medical personnel. Well done.

Perhaps on Tuesday you can ask the doctors what these events meant in the progression of the disease. Did the sudden explosion of fecal and urine material indicate that his elimination process is the result of a muscular failure, or inactivity due to constant sitting in the chair? In any case it was a surprising feature in Bob's long endurance of this disease.

You did exceptionally well in this emergency and we all appreciate your love and care for Bob. God bless and strengthen you. Jim"

Sunday, 27 May

Things have been the same the last couple of days except for today. Bob was more alert, although he was very feisty at times. I think the doctor must have lowered his medication yesterday. His eyes were open, all of the way, which was most unusual for him. It was almost one of those days that you hear people speak of. The loved one, who is ill, has a very good day, almost like a miracle happens and the ill one dies the next day. If Bob should die tomorrow I would not be surprised at all. I am prepared for Bob to die soon, I think, but this was such an unusual situation today.

The doctor on call telephoned me yesterday and she was very informative about Bob's condition. The pneumonia is still there and is due to the aspiration difficulty that Bob has. I believe they call this aspiration pneumonia. The doctor will continue treating with antibiotics. I did ask her what the prognosis is in view of the fact that Bob is eating next to nothing and his other problems, which are many, considering the Parkinson's disease is in its final stage. The answer she gave me was "Grave," which was no surprise, but at least she was honest.

The meeting on Tuesday will probably not give us any additional information about Bob since a doctor, or the nurse practitioner, will not be at the meeting. It will be the staff people responsible for taking care of Bob.

Monday, 28 May

Bob was a little feisty today but the medication took care of him although he did not sleep the entire time I was there. Tonight was about the same until he was given his medication.

He was glad to see me both times I visited today. But tonight he was especially glad to see me. He tried to take off his shoes so I took him back to his room, and asked him if he wanted me to wash his feet etc... He said yes. I rolled up his pants and really soaped up his feet and legs good, rinsed them off, and put lotion on them. I then did the same thing with his hands and face and neck. He is so funny because he just sits back, relaxed and seems like he enjoys me doing this for him or else he feels so nice and clean that he is relaxed during this time. About this time, the aide came in and she had another nurse with her, they got him into bed, and she finished washing him, and got him very comfortable for the night. I sat in with him, in the dark, he called for me several times and I told him I was just going to sit with him until he went to sleep, which he eventually did. I am so sorry that Bob looks so frightened when the aides lift him into bed. I hug and kiss him while the aides finish up washing him. He is so afraid they will drop him and I try to reassure him that they are professionals and have never dropped anyone. It does take a few minutes for him to settle down when they are finished washing him etc. so I always stay for awhile to make sure he is settled down and asleep before I leave.

Bob did get a very good shave today from a man who is a Physical Therapist in this unit. Bob did look good today. He is always clean and his clothes ironed and fresh. I bring his laundry home each evening, when I return home, wash every-thing, iron his shirts, and have everything ready to take back over to him every three days. His pants have nice creases and are wash-and-wear and do not need any touch up with the iron. I do not like the laundry to add up so I find it easier just to put the things in to wash each evening.

Tomorrow, after the meeting with the caregivers, staff people, Don and I are going to go to the Funeral Home to see what will be necessary to take when the time comes. I remember there might be several checks necessary, one to open the grave site for the cemetery, and I think one for the liner that goes in the grave. There are several other questions I want to ask and I would rather not wait until later, when it will probably be a very emotional time, to get some answers to my questions. I think I have everything in my mind as to what Bob and I decided we wanted to happen on the day of our funerals. Jim thinks I may have a negative attitude about Bob recovering. That is not the case. I know it will be soon and I am trying to be prepared so there are no surprises.

Tuesday, 29 May

All is the same today and tonight. Bob did eat for the nurse this evening and also earlier. He looks very good, although thin, which is natural since he isn't eating much.

We didn't learn anything new at the conference today. I guess speaking with the doctor on Saturday, when she called me after the episode on the lift, was good because I got an-swers to some of my questions. This doctor was not Bob's doctor but the doctor on call Friday night when the episode happened. She was very understanding and I liked speaking with her. Don said he thought the staff would do anything at all to help us, either for Bob or for me.

This evening, when I went back over, Bob was in bed sound asleep as they had given him his medication at 6pm and he goes to sleep in a few minutes after that. He was clean and comfortable and looked very peaceful.

I took one of the food supplements that Barbe had given me to help her dad sleep, last night about an hour before I went to bed and I had the best night's sleep in a long time. It was from about 11pm until 8am, when a telephone call awakened me. Otherwise I may still be asleep. It was a good night.

Don took me to the Funeral Home today that I was thinking of using later on down the road. The man that I wanted to see was not there but another man showed us around the different rooms. When we went to the door to enter the building, you had to ring a bell to enter, which I thought was not good. It looked to me like there could be trouble in the area which would be bad for parking there at night and asking people to do the same if they had to worry about their cars while in the Funeral Home. I will have the visitation in the chapel, where we live, and it will not be necessary for anyone to go to the Funeral Home, which is really in a bad area now.

I am still having a problem of how to handle the reception after the funeral. If we go to the cemetery, before the reception, I am sure people living outside of where we have our apartment will not return for the reception. Jim said the Funeral Home kept granddad until after the reception and they brought the casket back, picked up the people, and then went to the cemetery, which I remember. It seems like it will be difficult to laugh and visit with people and then go to the cemetery to finish the funeral. I will have to think about this some more and then decide how to handle the reception.

Wednesday, 30 May

Bob had a very good day today. One of the aides walked by. She thought he was sleeping and said, "Hi Mr. Awalt." Bob opened his eyes, smiled at her and waved to her. She was very surprised, as I was. He ate well at lunch time for the Director of this unit, ate ice cream for me and then ate a chocolate sundae for me. Naturally, he ate nothing at four o'clock. He really enjoyed his ice cream as Jim and I did also.

Tonight he was peaceful and sound asleep in bed when I returned to visit. I kissed him several times goodnight but he was in a deep sleep and did not awaken. I sat with him for awhile and then brought his laundry home to wash. The nurse said she was going to awaken him about nine to see if she could get him to eat a little.

I found the information on the internet about the Trappist Caskets which I remember Jim speaking about after attending a funeral for a friend of his. The caskets look very beautiful in their hand-rubbed simplicity. I am sure Bob would admire one of these if he saw it. He worked with restoring furniture and would always hand rub the wood and make it so beautiful. I remember how he rubbed and rubbed the fireplace wall in our living room where we lived before moving to our apartment. I am seriously thinking this type of casket would be so appropriate for a man like Bob who would also appreciate the thinking behind the monks making the caskets.

Thursday, 31 May

This has been another pretty good day for Bob. I received a telephone call from the Medical Center that the nurses found him on the pad on the floor next to his bed, which was in the lowest position. Therefore, if he fell out of bed onto the pad, it wasn't very far to drop. He was on his knees so he probably just slipped off of his bed. He was not hurt. In fact, he had a shower and a nice shave and really looked good. I do wish he felt as good as he looks. He also ate his lunch very well. He drank two glasses of apple juice and one glass of lemonade also.

Sunday, 03 June

I am very thankful that I was able to attend the sixtieth anniversary of the Ordination of Bob's brother, Bill, yesterday in Potomac, Maryland. Msgr. William J. Awalt is semi-retired from his priestly duties now. Our marriage was the next week or so after he was ordained in 1947. It has always meant a lot for Bob and me to remember that our marriage was the first for Msgr. Awalt to perform. He did a good job! Our son picked me up at the Medical Center, where I spent three hours with Bob, and we drove over to Potomac, Maryland to Our Lady of Mercy Church, for the Celebration Mass and reception for Bob's older brother's 60th Anniversary of his Ordination. I gave Don's cell phone number to the nurses to use in case I was needed for any reason. All went well and there were no telephone calls. I am very thankful that I was able to go and stop in to see Bob when we returned. I was so glad I stopped in to see Bob. His eyes were wide open and I believe he was waiting for me. I sat on the bed and he held my hand very tightly for about a half hour and then he drifted off to a deep sleep. When I was sure he was in a deep sleep, I took his laundry and went home. He looked so clean, comfortable and peaceful, and with no pain.

Everything is about the same with Bob. One day he will eat two meals and maybe the next day or two he will eat three. I see it makes a difference to Bob who is helping to feed him. I notice when the Director or nurse is feeding him, Bob does seem to eat better. I have wondered if they do not have the responsibility of taking care of several residents, and are able to take more time with Bob. Today Bob was wide awake, for the third day in a row, when I went in to visit him. I could understand most of what he said. He asked me if he was improving and getting better. I told him yes except for his legs, which are dead weight and he is unable to control. I still massage his legs and exercise them everyday and in the evening to try and keep some life in his muscles. Most of the rest of the time, when I visit, we just sit and talk. Many times there is no conversation, we just sit and hold hands. Sometimes Bob pats my hand or knee when I am sitting next to him. When you have been married for almost sixty years there are many times when it is not necessary to speak words. There is a mutual understanding that goes beyond the expression of any words. I know he is so glad to see me and appreciates the care I have given him. I believe Bob is also beginning to understand why he is in the Medical Center, that I am physically unable to lift him now that he can't use his legs at all. This has to be the worst part of his illness when the Stranger continues to take control of Bob's mind and body. Or, as the professionals call it, Bob is in the last stages of Parkinson's disease.

Monday, 04 June

Bob was wide awake again today until about 3pm when the Sundowning started. He was still agitated at 4pm when the staff tried to get him to eat, which he refused. They tried later to get him to eat and he pushed all food away. He had eaten very well at breakfast and lunch. Earlier I gave him ice cream that he seemed to enjoy. When I went back tonight, he was very peaceful, sleeping in his bed. I kissed him several times and he did not awaken. He was in deep sleep because he had finally agreed to take his medication. He is so changeable. I am sure that I could not continue to care for him at home. He needs professional help to cope with this Sundowning.

Wednesday, 06 June

No different news. Today was not good for Bob. He ate very little and he had to have his medication. The Stranger got into his body early this morning and he was very agitated.

There was a nice picnic, outside, with music, played by Fancy Pants, with hot dogs, hamburgers, snowballs, fruit, root beer floats etc... I cut up a hot dog in very small pieces and Bob ate them and seemed to enjoy them very much. He had not eaten anything since 7:30am this morning. The Fancy Pants band was very good but loud. I took Bob out but he wanted to leave because the music was too loud. I then took him over to the benches outside of the entrance and we could hear the music better; Bob fell asleep in the sun for about a half hour. I then took him inside and he continued to sleep for about another hour when Jim came over to see him.

Tonight I went back at 6pm and Bob was sound asleep in bed. He was clean and comfortable and looked very peaceful. I stayed with him for about an hour and then brought the wash home to do. I kissed him goodnight and as usual he did not wake up. I spoke for a few minutes with Larry and his mother Ann. She is such a sweet lady. I also spoke with Fred and Mary before leaving. There is so much sadness at the Medical Center that I just look around and give thanks for the good life Bob and I have had for almost sixty years. We enjoyed very good health for most of this time and not many couples can say this.

Thursday, 07 June

The day was very good for Bob. He ate three meals today all by himself, without the help of any of the aides. He was the talk of the whole place. He was anxious and agitated at times and asked all kinds of questions. He kept telling everyone that I was supposed to be there at 10am. Usually I get over to visit with Bob at twelve or a few minutes before or after. Today, I got over there early at fifteen minutes before twelve. When I got off of the shuttle, four aides got on the shuttle, going to lunch, and told me that Bob had been asking for me all morning etc...

I got back over to see him at five o'clock this evening after leaving at ten minutes before 4pm, and he was still up. I began to wash his feet, legs, arms and hands, face and even his teeth, which I was able to brush very well. He seemed to love the attention and he smelled so good from the lotion. He also helped the two aides, slightly, get him into bed.

The doctor saw Bob today and I was able to see him and speak with him. He said all is better with Bob. He said there are two types of people who enter the Long Term Care and they usually die of congestive heart failure. The first type die within a month or two, from congestive heart failure, and the second type usually live on for two or three years if their hearts are good. He said Bob falls into this second group because his heart is good except for a skipped beat or so, once in awhile. He also said he could "sugar coat" the prognosis but he didn't believe in doing that. I thanked him for his honesty. Bob still has some difficulty swallowing but it isn't too bad at this time. He ate chicken tonight that was cut up small but not ground up. Bob still has the aspiration pneumonia but it is not apparent all of the time when he eats or drinks. They have not needed the suction machine in the last two weeks. I believe a lot of his problems must have been associated with the medication Bob was given to get him to calm down and to resist the Stranger, who was trying to get into his mind and body.

I also asked the doctor if he felt that Bob would ever be controlled with a maintenance amount of medication, and return to his home. He said absolutely not. He said he still has the last stages of Parkinson's disease even though it may last a long time. I asked him also when Bob gets agitated in the morning if it means the Sundowning is starting earlier in the day. He said yes it does, and also some residents there become agitated just by sitting around everyday. This is why they try to get them to play bingo and some of the other games. It looks like Bob will be condemned to sit in his chair forever. This is a long chair, similar to a wheel chair, only it is more like a chaise lounge that can be raised or lowered and rolled around. This is a terrible sentence for someone who has always been such a good person and so active. The Parkinson's disease and the Stranger have finally succeeded in taking over Bob's mind and body completely.

Friday, 08 June

Bob did very well with his meals today by eating all of them by himself, with no help from the aides. He was still awake when I went back tonight so I did my usual chores, which seem to please both of us, and the aides got him into bed, after they finished washing him. He was asleep when I left and looked very peaceful. The aides do a nice job of finishing up washing Bob and getting him to bed. Bob is still frightened, by the terrifying look in his eyes, thinking they will drop him. I keep telling Bob they are professionals and work very quickly. I worked much slower when I helped him before he moved into the Medical Center because I didn't want to hurt him. I often told him I wish he could understand what good care he was getting and to try not to be afraid. I also tried to help him understand that I was right with him every night to make sure he wasn't hurt and even to help the aides if necessary. It didn't help Bob at all; he was still frightened.

Saturday, 09 June

Today was an entirely different story for Bob. In the first place, when I went in to visit with him, at 8:30am, I noticed he had the "wrap around vest with the two long metal stays" which was accidentally left behind Bob's back, in the chair that he is confined to sit in now. I can't imagine anything worse than sitting against these two metal stays for ten or twelve hours with those stays digging into your back. I quickly approached two aides to come over and help get the garment from behind Bob's back. They came over and removed the vest that is used with the lift to help Bob to be removed from the chair into the bed or lifted from the bed onto the chair.

I was also told Bob would not eat anything for his lunch until the nurse fixed him an egg sandwich, which she put into his hand and he did eat. When the nurse brought over his medication, he spit it out. Later I asked him if he wanted to take his medication so he could improve, and he finally agreed. When the nurse came over the second time, with the medication, Bob did hesitate opening his mouth, for her to put the medicine in, but she finally got it in. The staff has a lot of patience in taking care of the residents especially when they are giving out the medications.

For the rest of the day that I was with Bob, he was very agitated. The vest, when left in the chair behind Bob's back, was very painful and adds to his agitation. He tried to get out of the chair from twelve o'clock until three forty-five when I planned on going over to eat my dinner. I noticed his face was getting very red and very hot. The aide finally took his temperature which was somewhat high. He had just worked so hard trying to get out of the chair that he was making himself sick. They put an ice pack in back of his neck to cool him down. This was so close to the evening meal, I knew he would not eat as he was too upset. He finally did eat the ice cream from inside a cone. I do not give him the cone because I am afraid he may have trouble swallowing the pieces.

I took Bob to his room after I gave him the ice cream, washed his feet and massaged his legs, hands, face, and teeth, and he did seem to calm down when he realized his was going to bed. The aide came in and said she would get the lift to put him into bed. When I explained the lift was not to be used anymore to help put Bob to bed, she went to get another aide to help her lift Bob onto the side of the bed. She proceeded to finish washing him and got him ready for bed.

Sunday, 10 June

Today was worse than yesterday. Among other things, Bob kicked one of the nurses in her back, which was already injured some time ago from helping another resident, and she left early. I did see her and she looked like she was in pain. They finally gave Bob a needle, with his medication. It finally worked and he slept for about two hours.

When he awakened, he ate an ice cream sandwich and drank a small glass of cranberry juice. This is all he had to eat all day. Jim came back to give Bob Holy Communion since he had been asleep earlier. Later, it was apparent the medication was wearing off and I could foresee trouble this evening when I return to visit with Bob.

Bob was calm tonight. He did not eat any dinner again. When I got over there tonight, the two aides were finishing up getting him into bed and he was clean and comfortable. I sat with him for an hour and he slept very peacefully. He said a few things that I could not understand. It was almost like he was talking in his sleep.

The two aides said all had gone well in getting him ready and into bed. The one aide was just finishing up wiping his wheel chair all over and even shined up the chrome. They were unusually good workers.

The staff gives Bob a little time, when he acts up; to make sure he doesn't need an increase in the medication. This is good because sometimes when I get there he settles down and will cooperate and may need less medication. The less medication he has the better everyone can understand his speech, or so it seems. I will see what happens tomorrow.

Monday, 11 June

Bob was in bed at noon today for a nap, when I got over to see him. He had asked to go to bed. He said he was tired. He did not eat any food at all. He awakened after sleeping for a couple of hours. Don came over to see him and Bob awakened and knew Don was there.

When we were getting ready to leave, I called the aides to get Bob out of bed to go to the dining room for his dinner. I knew he would not eat in bed. He hasn't so far. They brought in the lift, with the hammock, and asked me if I had seen it before. I said no and we just waited to see how it works. It is the safest thing to get Bob out of bed. It is better than two people pulling on him. Don clapped his hands when they finished because it worked so well. They promised the pad would be removed immediately, which it was. I am very glad I was able to see how it worked. This lift, with the hammock, is entirely different than the lift which the patient has to stand on and hold on.

Bob was clean and comfortable tonight in bed when I returned. He ate nothing for dinner except a couple of spoons full of soup and a small amount of cranberry juice. This was all he had to eat or drink today. He would not take any ice cream or apple juice from me either. He was sleeping in his chair so they put him into bed early. He did awaken once and I think he knew I was there. I sat with him for a little more than an hour in case he awakened again, which he did not.

Tuesday, 12 June

Got some good news!!!! I asked the aides today to give Bob some Seafood Newburg over a helping of mashed potatoes tonight for his dinner. I waited, with Jim, until it was time to take Bob in for his dinner. The servers in the dining room asked me again for suggestions for Bob to eat and I told them the same thing. Well, they brought out his plate and it looked so good with all these shrimp, scallops, cream sauce, and over these fortified mashed potatoes with a glass of milk and a roll. Well, he started to eat, by himself, immediately and really enjoyed it all. I said to Jim that it was wonderful to see this happening. He was a sight for sore eyes. I think he just didn't like the ground up food.

I sent an email to the doctor and asked him if he didn't think Bob could handle regular food now. He has good teeth and he always chewed his food very well. I did not wait for his okay however. When I got home tonight I received an email from him telling me that he would order a regular menu for Bob. Great!!

This doctor has been so wonderful in dealing with me by email. He knew I could not always get to the telephone, so he would email messages to me. This was great because many times it was 2am-3am before I could respond to him but I was always able to do so in a timely manner.

The Director had told me that before Bob could have regular food they would have to bring in the Speech Therapist to check his swallowing. I told the doctor, by email, that Bob was eating Ice cream sandwiches without any trouble and I didn't believe he needed the ground food anymore.

At any rate, he may not be able to handle some things but I believe he can handle most food. He never was one to prefer a steak or something like that.

His medication has been increased a little and you can tell when it wears off. But, at least, he may get some pleasure from his food. He was very restless in bed tonight after the aides finished getting him ready and in bed. Finally, I asked him to give up, roll over and go to sleep, which he did. I sat with him for awhile, he called me several times to see if I was still there, I went over and kissed him a couple of times and off to sleep he went. I do hope he has a good night.

I saw Larry and his mother, Ann, again and I just have to remark what a sweet lady she is. She has the most beautiful complexion for anyone her age, or for that matter, any age. Larry is the youngest of her four children and he is so devoted. He comes every evening to visit with her. She will open her eyes and smile when he is there with her. They really must have a special bond, this mother and son.

Wednesday, 13 June

This is a copy of an email I sent to Bob's new doctor this evening. His wonderful doctor has left the area and moved to Florida to be nearer his family. My heart almost broke when he left.

I was so upset when I came home that I could hardly speak to anyone, much less the nice lady that I enjoy seeing every night. She is one of the people who completes my day when I can visit with her, even if it is for a short while.

"I realize Bob needs the medication, at times, to calm him down. Tonight, just when he was beginning to eat his dinner, the staff member gave him this medication as he was agitated and trying to get out of his chair. The medication knocked him out so fast that I called the nurse practitioner over to check him. His eyes rolled back into his head and he almost looked like he was going into shock or a coma. She didn't think there was a problem. I took him back to his room, washed his hands and face and he seemed to slip further away making sounds like he could not get his breath. The aide came into his room to get him ready for bed and asked if he was normally like this. I asked her to take his blood pressure, which she did, and it was 60/44. He was totally unresponsive. She went to get help and a nurse and the aides came in and said this was the way the medication was supposed to work.

The aides got him into bed, and finished up. I sat with him for about an hour to make sure he was sleeping and breathing normally, which he was. This does seem to be a drastic way of addressing this situation. Or, could he have a reaction to this medication?

Thank you for your attention in this matter."

It seems to me there should be a better way of handling a situation like this. No doubt Bob is agitated at times and does need medication. I can't understand why it has to be so drastic. I will see what Bob's new doctor has to say in the morning.

Wednesday, 13 June — Later

I just received a telephone call from the Medical Center; the aide told me the aide found Bob on the floor in his room. The medication had worn off and he had fallen out of bed onto the pad on the floor. He did not get hurt. This is the third time it has happened. It must have happened in his sleep or else he didn't try to walk. Thank goodness or he would have been hurt if he would have fallen on the hard floor. When I left tonight the aide told me that she would keep an eye on him, which she did. I am glad I didn't go back again tonight; it would have been too upsetting.

Friday, 15 June

Not much news tonight. Bob ate a good brunch today, and a cup of ice cream for me this afternoon. He ate nothing to-night and was really agitated. He let me do the wash up, what I do each night, but gave the aides a hard time when they tried to take his shirt off tonight. He finally went to sleep still agitated with me, because I let the aide take care of him. I sat with him for awhile to make sure he was in a deep sleep and not faking. I thought he was sleeping soundly. So, I will see what happens tomorrow. I still could hear some congestion and his voice was raspy, kind of like a foghorn at times.

Saturday, 16 June

Good news tonight about Bob. He ate very well at the brunch and dinner times. I got over there today, just when it was time to order his food. He would not or could not answer the server so I ordered a bowl of crab soup, mashed potatoes, peas, and one half hot turkey sandwich and cranberry juice with orange juice for him. I held the soup bowl up so he could scoop up the soup more easily, which he ate every drop, and then I held up his dinner plate and he really ate like he was starved. He enjoyed every bit of his meal. Boy, you should have seen the crab soup which was loaded with crab meat and veggies. Then at twelve o'clock they gave him his medication and he fell off to sleep for almost two hours. When he awakened I gave him a cup of chocolate ice cream.

Tonight I got over just as he was finished his meal and was finishing his ice cream. Same thing, they gave him his medication and he fell off to sleep. I took him in his room, washed his feet and legs, hands and face and even got to clean his teeth real good. He awakened just as I finished his teeth. He is so used to me cleaning his teeth that he will open his mouth wide for me to brush his teeth, even if he is asleep. I love taking care of him or at least doing what I can to help him be more comfortable. I do not want him to have a toothache now with all of the other problems he now has.

The aide finished up after she and another aide got him into bed. I sat with him for about an hour and was sure he was sound asleep and then came home to do his laundry, which isn't much, but I prefer doing it nightly to keep it from getting ahead of me. He looks very peaceful, clean and comfortable. I have complete "peace of mind" until I get another call that he has fallen out of bed again.

It is now 10:20pm and the telephone call, from the Medical Center, just came in again. Bob had fallen out of bed and the alarm had alerted the staff and they found him on the floor in his room. He was not hurt and they got him back into bed and hopefully he will sleep the night through.

Monday, 18 June

Today was awful! The staff is trying to work with Bob. This morning was a disaster! This afternoon went better until it was time for Bob's dinner. Bob did not want me to leave for anything. I was fifteen minutes late meeting Jim for dinner and when I got there he was on the phone, calling all around trying to find me. He had just left Bob and me twenty minutes earlier.

Bob was really agitated in the dining room. The Director had helped get Bob to a table and picked out the food for his dinner. He was pushed all the way under the table and he could not move. I am so sorry but I continue to wonder if Bob gets agitated because I leave him to go and eat dinner and then return to visit with him. I do this so he won't depend on me entirely to help him eat. Many times he has eaten much better for a staff member than he will eat for me. I do believe the Stranger, in Bob's mind and body, doesn't miss an opportunity to upset him.

I ate hurriedly and rushed back over at 5pm and found he had eaten a very good dinner with the Director. The staff member then gave Bob his medication and I took him back to his room. The aides all came up to me and said to be sure and ring for help if I needed help with Bob back in his room, which I didn't think I would need. I did wonder if Bob had really given them a bad time and had been very agitated fighting the Stranger.

We got to his room and I asked him if he wanted me to start to take off his shoes and wash his legs, feet, hands and arms, and face. He looked at me and said yes. So, I began and I really dragged it out a long time and kept asking him if his legs felt better and he said yes. Finally, after I finished cleaning his teeth he fell asleep. The rest is history. The two aides came in, got him in bed, finished washing him and tucked him into his covers. I sat with him awhile to make sure he was sound asleep, which he was. Also, the aide put a wedge under the cover to keep him from rolling out of bed again.

I will get a glass of wine, try to read a little and then get ready for bed. Bob really tires me out when I have to talk so much to him to calm him down.

Tuesday, 19 June

Bob was very agitated again today, almost like the Stranger is trying to take over Bob's mind and body earlier and earlier. After eating nothing all day, I did get Bob to eat an ice cream sandwich. This evening at 4pm I left him to be helped with his eating but I think he was so agitated he would eat nothing. He had tried, from twelve noon until I left at five minutes before 4pm, to get out of his chair. Jim was there and even said he feels so sorry for Bob that he can't just accept that he is there. I know the staff had not given him the medication he needed to calm him down but they were trying to wait until after dinner. After I got over there at 5pm, the nurse tried four times to give it to him and he spit it out each time. They will not force him to eat or take medication. If he gets too bad the staff will give him medication in a needle in his hand or by liquid in the front of his mouth, under his tongue.

Bob continued to be very agitated when I took him to his room. I did the usual routine, which does seem to calm him somewhat. I dragged the rubbing of his legs and feet, hands and arms, and face out as long as I could. I was able to also clean his teeth, which I did, without asking him. I was then able to get one of the aides, who has had good luck with Bob, and told her I was ready with him and that he really wanted to go to bed. When she saw that I had even taken his shirt off and had his night shirt on, she called for help and the two aides got him into bed. He was peaceful, clean and comfortable and went right off to sleep. I sat with him for awhile and then brought the wash home. I hope he continued to sleep for the night but I doubt it. The aide also put the piece of foam and a pillow next to him, under the bottom sheet, to prevent him rolling out of bed. I hope it works. I know they are trying very hard to help him, and at times it couldn't be easy, and I also know they are used to helping this type of patient. They always tell me this is typical of Parkinson's patients who are in the last stages of the disease.

I keep wondering if Bob becomes more agitated with me because I leave him to go eat dinner. I do return by 5pm, which isn't long to take for dinner. I try to go to dinner most days so I can keep up my strength and be of more help to Bob when I go to visit. Jim and I eat dinner with Bob one night a week to keep him company. He is very hard to figure out.

Wednesday, 20 June

I met with the Director today and everything is worked out fine. I had a long talk with her and just kept to the facts. She is very nice and is trying hard to work with Bob. I know it isn't easy when he is spitting out his medicine and carrying on. They are doing their best to get the medication leveled out to a point that will keep Bob comfortable but under control. This has been very frustrating to me and to Bob because he has never had any medication that he did not have bad side effects from. I am sure Bob feels the difference the medication makes in his system. I just wish the Stranger would ease up and let Bob have a peaceful end.

The nurse came in and gave Bob one type of medication, just as he was moved into position at the table to eat his dinner. His eyes just stared at the ceiling in a fixed position for about three or four minutes, which seemed like such a long time. Then his eyes rolled back in his head and he appeared to pass out. Thank goodness he was in the long wheel chair. I kept talking to him but he was completely unresponsive. He did not change color this time. Finally, after what seemed a long time, Bob started to regain consciences and I was able to help him eat a little of his dinner. The whole affair took almost two hours before we finished what he could eat and leave the dining room at six o'clock. We had entered the dining room for dinner at 4pm.

The rest of the evening was uneventful except when the nurse tried to give Bob his next medication; he spit it out four times. I took Bob back to his room, washed him, as I usually do, and the aide came in with the machine that lifts Bob into bed. I tried to reassure Bob the aide will work quickly and for him to not be afraid. I told him that this was a very safe machine. This machine has a hammock to sit on and the patient does not stand. The aide can get him into bed quickly and easily with this machine and without the help of another aide. I waited and sat with Bob for a while, to make sure he was asleep, which he was and then left. He looked very peaceful and comfortable. I hope he has a good night.

Thursday, 21 June

Jim had a nice dinner with Bob tonight. Bob ate very well at the brunch time, for one of our favorite aides, after he had his shower, shaved really well and she even tried to use an emery board on his nails. I did finish his nails when I was there. Tonight Bob ate everything on his plate, salmon cake, macaroni and cheese, stewed tomatoes, plus one and a half bowls of soup, skim milk, and finished off with an ice cream sandwich. Wow!!! He even scraped his dish and got all of the juice from the stewed tomatoes.

When the aide took his blood pressure late today, when Jim and I were with him at almost 4pm, it was 84 over 54. Not too good!!! The aide that took the blood pressure was facing me, and she asked me if I saw his blood pressure on the machine. Nothing more was said but she is the one who has been trying to alert me that Bob has many problems which are difficult to live with.

Today was our 60th wedding anniversary and I was with Bob most of the day. I told him of the flowers and the many cards which I showed him several times. He patted my hand several times and gave me some kisses and his love. It almost breaks my heart to see him in this condition and yet not let him see how miserable I am for him.

The staff put a notice in his room, signed by the three aides who helped give him his shower, which I was glad to see. It said "Mr. Awalt had shower at 9:30am today" and it was signed by the three aides that helped give it to him. He also had his hair washed. I wrote on the bottom of it "Thank you very much." I hope they took the message that I was thanking them for giving him the shower and for putting the notice up for me. I have more peace of mind for Bob when I am told all that goes on toward his care and comfort. Yes, I am particular but that is what he is used to.

Actually, this was another one of those days that if Bob dies tomorrow or so I will be one of those people who say what a good day he had today. I believe at this point that his blood pressure will probably get lower and lower. I am sure this is why he wants to get back into bed so early, in fact, right after he eats his dinner. Jim noticed the change in the skin color of his hands today. He said it was probably due to the low blood pressure.

After Jim left I finished washing his hands, face, legs and feet for him. I also put the nice lotion on them and he seems content except for wanting to get right into bed. We waited for the nurse to bring his medicine to him and then the two aides came to his room and put him into bed. He didn't go right off to sleep as he usually does but after a short while he was sound asleep. Bob did not have the Stranger trying to control him tonight. This makes such a difference in his behavior but I know this Stranger will not give up until he has complete control over Bob's mind and body.

I am glad I decided to go ahead and order his casket from the Trappist Monks. They will just keep it in storage until it is needed. It makes no difference how long a period of time this may be. When the casket is needed, they will ship it in two days. If it is needed before the two day period, they guarantee it can be delivered by the time it is needed. It is going to be handmade from beautiful Walnut wood; hand-rubbed to a beautiful finish and will have a small cross on top. When the Trappist Monks make these caskets they also pray a lot and put so much feeling into making them. I was really impressed and sincerely believe Bob would admire the work that has gone into making the casket. Bob did so much work with wood and especially hand-rubbing the wood until it was just the way he wanted it. It was never too much trouble for him to rub many times before he was finally satisfied and finished what he was working on.

Friday, 22 June

It is now 9am and no telephone calls from the Medical Center as yet. I waited until 2pm and had not received any call then. Bob was so much on my mind that it was very difficult to sleep. I have decided to stay over with him today, at the dinner time also, because I do not have the heart to leave him to get my dinner and then return to finish my visit with him. I will see if I am right or wrong now about the end of suffering for Bob to be over soon.

Friday, 22 June

I am including an email from Bob's brother to me because I believe it expresses some of my own thoughts, especially when I am helping Bob to eat. He also voices some concerns for me. I keep telling him that I am fine. Yes, I do wish that I could still take care of Bob completely but I know he needs professional help to get him through these last stages of Parkinson's disease. This email was an answer to one that I had sent to Jim canceling dinner for tonight.

"I understand and we will miss you. You seem however to have changed to a more pessimistic view about Bob's ability to survive. Did something new occur? I know this daily care is taking a toll on you, particularly in your emotional/mental response. Is it possible to for you to talk to or seek some one (lay or professional) to evaluate your schedule with Bob? My new insight from last night's dinner (and this is my amateur opinion) is he is operating at a lower mental measure. I don't know what part the medication has on this but you said that another medication was due after supper, so I would presume the last dose was weakening as a deterrent in his behavior. But the events that stood out for me were (positive points) that he was alert to us at least to notice us with eyes open. He is able to feed himself when he is given the right utensil and has no difficulty in filling it. He has great strength and fine body organ function. This would seem to say his body is strong for some time to come. Unless there is some heart, respiratory or kidney outbreak I would conclude that his longevity is good. (Negatively) He won't be a happy patient because he does not want to be there. He has an obsession in him that motivates him all the time even while he eats with us; going along the corridors. This obsession overrides his own mind and advice you give to him. At supper the negative things I observed that don't measure up to his other positive points are a complete ignorance of basic moves. He doesn't identify spoon from knife, he is not aware until the food touches his mouth or is given to him what it is he desires. Concentration on removing crumbs or perceived crumbs overtakes any other function. I say this with a sad heart, I couldn't suppress the thought that I was present at the feeding of a small child. My presence I felt was important to hopefully to give him some sense that I still love him as a brother. But it saddens me to believe this may go on for some time. I pray for him ardently, but I am also concerned that this schedule you keep may affect you. I know that your love pushes you this way. But perhaps others who know such situations from experience or training may shed some understanding for you."

Friday, 22 June — Later

Yesterday was a good day. When I arrived at the Medical Center, for my visit, Bob was at the nurse's station telling one of the nurses about the Baltimore Gas & Electric Company's Crane Station and the details of when he was working. I asked him if he remembered when the station was built and when we attended the grand opening. He said, "Yes, and butt out." Haha—It was so funny. The aides remarked they had never heard Bob speak of his working in business before and they couldn't believe how good his memory was.

The aides told me Bob had eaten well except he did not want his ice cream so one of the aides would bring it to me about 1pm, which she did. In fact, he kept opening his mouth for more ice cream sandwich, after eating one, that I went back and got another and he ate the entire second ice cream sandwich.

After he had his medicine, 12pm, eaten his ice cream sand-wiches, he went to sleep, in the chair, until Jim came over at 2:30pm. Jim left at three twenty-five, to catch the shuttle at three thirty, and Bob went back to sleep until I left about three fifty to go over and eat dinner. I left Bob at the nurse's station so they could keep an eye on him.

After dinner, when I returned at 5pm, Bob was in the din-ing room with an aide trying to feed him. He wouldn't eat a thing, which was meat loaf, mashed potatoes, etc.; and he would only keep trying to swing the table around. He was very agitated. I took him back to his room and tried to calm him down. Finally, after telling him how hungry he was going to be later, I asked him if he wanted a meat loaf sandwich. He said yes, so back we went to the dining room. They fixed him a good one half of meat loaf sandwich, which I asked for, and I gave him a glass of apple juice and he really went to town eating it. We went back to his room and he insisted on getting into bed. I washed his feet, legs, hands and face and usually this is very relaxing for him. He kept insisting he wanted to get into bed. I told him the aides would be along shortly but he had to wait his turn. The aide came in with the lift, which works like a hammock that you sit in, and she was able to get him into bed very quickly. Then he started fighting her to try and stop her from taking off his pants. She tried to explain that his wife took his clothes home each night to wash them. It didn't work at all. He was fighting for his life. He kept putting his legs out of the bed, to get up. When the aide finally released his grip, on her arms, I blocked his legs, and she went for help. She couldn't call this time because all of the aides were helping others.

The aide came back with three aides and they put Bob back in his wheelchair and also placed the tray on it, which really blocks him into the chair. They asked me when I left if I would bring him back to the nurse's station so they could watch him, which I did. In the meantime, I pushed the chair up and down the halls to try and calm him down. He was still so agitated that he tried to reach for any and everything he could to grab hold of to stop us. After an hour and a half of walking and pushing him and making sure we would walk in the very middle of the hall, so he could not reach anything to grab, I took him back to the nurse's station. I stayed there with him for a while and several people came over to speak to him, including Larry. Bob answered him and spoke to him very calmly. I wasn't sure if the second dose of medicine was taking effect or he was getting exhausted. After another short while I told him I would see him in the morning and I left. I knew there was no damage he could do to hurt himself or others at that point. I saw the aide as I left and she told me she would put him to bed later and please not to worry. In fact, she said for me to telephone the desk if I wanted to have more peace of mind later on. I told her I would not call as I had every confidence they would handle the situation well. I did not call.

I had a nice drink of wine, read the mail, got ready for bed and slept like a log as I was so tired. I knew one of the staff would call me if Bob fell or anything happened. One thing stands out in my mind; as much as I would love to have Bob home to care for, I could not handle him when he has the Sundowning take over his mind and body. It takes several people to work with him and even then they are not successful.

Saturday, 23 June

I just got home from visiting with Bob, about 9:30pm. Today was very good, with Bob eating very well for me. He had cream chipped beef on a biscuit, juice, etc. at lunch time and finished it all like he hadn't eaten in a week. He also finished up with his ice cream sandwich.

Tonight he had veal parmesan, which was such a large portion he only ate half of it, with a large scoop of mashed potatoes, roll and a half-and-half drink, which is half orange juice and half cranberry juice. He also finished up with his ice cream sandwich.

Both times tonight, when I was feeding him, he slumped over in his chair, completely unresponsive, eyes back in his head, etc... But each time it only lasted a few seconds, maybe a minute and he was OK. After a short while he continued to eat and finally finished.

The staff kept Bob in the chair all day, with the tray on it, to keep him from getting out. They are also putting him to bed at 10pm tonight so he will go to sleep and stay there. I took him back to his room and washed his legs and feet, hands and face, and even his teeth tonight. Then, I put his nightshirt on him and wheeled him back down to the nurse's station for them to watch him until they put him to bed at ten. He waved me off when I left and he seemed to finally accept the situation, almost like he was giving in to the Stranger.

Wednesday, 27, June

Bob is just the same. When he has the medication working he is good. When the medication wears off, he is a terror. One exception: yesterday morning the activities director had him playing wheelchair basketball. She couldn't get over the strength he has in his arms to throw the ball across the room and into the hoop. I think he was the only one who got most of the balls into the basket. I think the mornings are a little better for him.

I am staying over until about 9pm now because they have found if he goes to bed later, he sleeps through the night and doesn't get out of bed. The staff has three alarms on Bob, one on his cover, one on the bed, and the other on the floor with an eye to sound off when he either gets out of bed or falls out of bed.

I still get him ready, wash up and complete my chores and then take him back to the nurse's station where they can watch him. He doesn't like it at all. He wants to go to bed but this is the only way to keep him from getting hurt. The night before last he was wide awake until 1:30am before he got tired enough to sleep. Most of the time, he was trying to get out of the chair. When he is like that, the nurses put the tray back on so he can't get out and just wait for him to tire himself out enough to sleep through the night.

When I get home, I am tired and put the wash in, get ready for bed and jump in. I don't get to sleep right away but I do try to rest for the next day.

Thursday, 28 June

This was a bad day for Bob. Nothing went right for him. He was agitated very early in the day. Sometimes I really wonder why. He only ate half of a sandwich for the noonday meal and no ice cream, which is most unusual. Jim and I were still with him at 4pm when the nurse gave him his medication. I knew this must be wrong but I said nothing. I went home and checked my notes and found the order had been changed two weeks ago that the staff was not to give Bob any medication right before a meal. When I went back over, after dinner, there was Bob sound asleep and not a bit of his dinner was he able to eat. I really fussed at the nurse who had given him this medication. Two and one half hours later, she came over, tried her best to awaken Bob and gave him a vanilla milkshake and I finally got him to eat half of a ham sandwich with a small glass of Coke.

Friday, 29 June

Today was very good for Bob. I am not sure if they have adjusted his medication to a level that makes him calm or it was just a good day. He ate very well, on his own, without help, and he also ate a container of yogurt and drank a small container of chocolate milk. After dinner tonight he was a real terror. The Stranger was in his body and really took hold of him. Bob begged me to have the tray removed that was preventing him from getting out of the chair and hurting himself. He said he was grateful for all of the help I had given him, and this almost made the tears flow. I kept telling him that if he could stop being so angry, the tray would be removed. It was just awful to see him suffer like this and I am unable to help him.

When I left him, after washing his feet and legs, arms and hands, and face and teeth, he continued to fight me all the way, which was very unusual, I asked him for a kiss good-night. He said only a small one because I did not help him get out of the chair, which is really sad. I keep telling him that only nurses can unlock the tray and remove it when he calms down. He said he was very sorry he lost his temper. I do wish he was strong enough to get rid of the Stranger before he has complete control over his mind and body.

I am so glad I was able to give him a good haircut earlier today. The two aides had really given him a good shower and a wonderful shave with a regular razor, not the electric razor. They do a great job. I have told the one aide repeatedly that she is going to make a very good nurse. Bob looked so good and I told him again that I did wish he could have felt better because he looked so good.

I was speaking with two of the staff about something, when the conversation turned to the identification bracelets, which I asked them about again. They said all people there should have one and I told them both that Bob has never had one in the two months that he has been there. They both indicated this would be corrected. I looked around, when I was over at the Medical Center this evening, and found very few people had an identification bracelet on. I can only guess they probably removed their bracelets.

Sunday, 01 July

Today was a very good day for Bob. The staff at the Medical Center did not need to put the tray across Bob's lap to keep him from getting out or falling out of the chair. This evening was a different story because he was so agitated. He worked for a long time trying to get out of his chair, and he almost succeeded in climbing out of the chair a couple of times.

Later I took Bob to his room and did the wash-up chores that I like to do for him each night, and he was still highly agitated. He did help me take off his shirt and put on the nightshirt. When I was leaving, I took him back to the nurse's station for them to keep an eye on him as he was too agitated to go to bed. The nurses keep him up, watching him, until he appears to be getting very sleepy. I asked him if he wanted to give me a kiss goodnight, which he did very quickly, and said goodnight. I hope the medication was finally taking effect so he could have a good night of sleep.

Monday, 02 July

Today was about the same for Bob. He did eat well this evening but not this morning. I asked if he had been given his medication when he awakened early and the answer was yes. Naturally, he was in a deep sleep. I was able to awaken him enough for him to drink a half glass of juice and eat half of a hot dog and one teaspoon of baked beans. About two-thirty, when Bob was awake, I gave him a rather large container of peach yogurt and he drank a small box of chocolate milk. I am sure he ate well tonight as all of the food on his plate was gone and there was evidence that he had eaten his ice cream sandwich.

It is a very sad situation when Bob looks at me and tells me that he loves me, appreciates what I have done for him and is grateful and then says, "Can't you help me now?" There is nothing more I can do for him except watch and make sure that he gets the best care possible. The Medical Center where he is is still the best for care that I have heard of or seen. Jim and both of our children agree to this. However, it doesn't make it any easier when Bob wants to come home so much. It breaks my heart!

Tuesday, 03 July

This was a good day for Bob. He ate well at two of his meals and was very glad to see me. After dinner he would not take his medication, and when I finally got one spoonfull in his mouth he spit it out all over his clothes. I took him to his room and did the usual chores, which I call the wash-up, and shortly after I finished the two aides came in to finish up and get him into bed. He was like a wild man, and it took three of us to hold him down for the aides to finish up washing him and getting him ready for bed. I sat with him, in the dark room, until nine thirty to see that he didn't get out of bed. He almost got out several times; so I told the nurses and they decided to put him back into his chair and take him back to the nurses' station until he settles down. It is no wonder he sleeps so much through the day. What is next? I certainly can't predict. The Stranger is working overtime trying to take complete control of Bob's mind and body. How much longer will it take before the Stranger wins?

Wednesday, 04 July

Today was pretty good for Bob. I have come to the conclusion that the early time of the day is much easier for Bob. He is in better spirits when it is early and before the Sundowning takes effect. I stayed over and ate dinner with Bob this evening although he was somewhat agitated. He did eat well considering all.

He was fit to be tied tonight when the nurse tried to give him his medication. This is the second night in a row that he would not take it. He even spit it out both nights. The nurse even tried to bribe him by telling him she would remove the tray, which is confining, if he would take it. He refused and when I did get a little in his mouth he would pick out the medicine that was ground up in apple sauce. I finally gave up after trying to get him to take his medicine for more than an hour. I asked him to remove his shirt, which had a mess on the front of it, from spitting up the medicine, which he did easily. I went to his room and got a nightshirt and put that on him. This is the first time in two months that I have not stayed long enough to wash his face, arms, hands, legs, and feet and then put the lotion on them. I feel awful about leaving him but he really tired me out. I am exhausted.

Thursday, 05 July

Today was a very changeable day for Bob. He did not eat well at either the morning breakfast or lunch time. I was able to give him some yogurt, in the afternoon, and an ice cream sandwich this evening. The nurse was unable to give him his medication so I asked her if I could try giving him the pills, instead of the pills ground up in pudding, and she agreed. This went well both times for Bob taking his medication. He was very calm and I was able to do the "wash up" chores in the late evening. At one point, he took my hand and kissed it about five times. This really breaks my heart to see him go through all of this frustration. After I washed him, I then took him up to the nurse's station, which he didn't like at all. I guess he thought he was going to bed, which was too early for him. He would only get out of bed and probably get hurt. I also asked the nurse to have the nurse practitioner look at Bob's legs again. They are swollen and the small cuts do not seem to heal. There are also more of them—almost like the skin is breaking down. When I left Bob was very agitated and trying like mad to get out of the chair, which he almost did. There were three aides standing near him trying to calm him down. I am so sorry to see him so upset before going to bed. It is no wonder he has bad dreams.

Friday, 06 July

Today was not a good day for Bob. When I got over to the

Care Center, Bob was in the reception room sound asleep in his long chair. The aides said that Bob had not gone into the dining room because he was asleep. I took him into the dining room and after many attempts finally was able to feed him a nice helping of cream chipped beef over toast. We went into the recreation room and he slept for two hours. When Jim came over, at three o'clock I took Bob's blood pressure and it continues to be very low, 77/48. It is no wonder his legs, feet, and one hand are very swollen. Bob told me he asked the aide not to put his shoes on when he was dressed and I can only guess because they felt tight.

When I returned to visit, after dinner, Bob was in the dining room feeding himself. He ate about half of his meal and he was finished. I am not sure if he stopped because I was there, and he wanted to leave, or if he was finished. I will never know. Later on, I did give him some ice cream and ginger ale. I was able to take him to his room and do my wash-up chores. He helped to take off his shirt and the outer shirt. When we were finished I took him back to the nurse's station, so they could watch him that he didn't fall out of his chair. My heart breaks when he looks at me so sad and he wanted to go to bed so badly. This is the first and only time he did not want to kiss me goodbye or even tell me goodbye. When he goes to bed before ten o'clock, he will sleep for a couple of hours and then get out of bed. I know he will only get hurt by doing this. I wish he could understand how awful it will be if he falls out of bed and gets a broken hip or some other bone. My heart aches for him to understand, which I know he can't handle.

I have sent an email to the nurse practitioner to see if I can get some answers to questions about his care. I just can't imagine they still have not given out identification bracelets to correctly identify the residents. I have witnessed the same questions being asked the residents, to identify themselves when some of them are not capable of doing this. It is so scary to see this and then wonder if Bob is getting his correct medication. This still looks to me like an accident about to happen. I will see what the nurse practitioner has to say when she answers my email, which will probably not be until Monday.

Saturday, 07 July

This evening turned out to be a very mixed-up affair. It was decided, by the aides, to get Bob ready for bed a little earlier than the previous night. This was because I asked them to so I could get his pants off of him, take them home with me to wash, since they had been on him for two days. I almost believe he slept in them. The aides had told me that he was very restless all night.

The aide brought in the lift machine, which requires the patient to stand on it and hold on. I said "No, that machine is not to be used." The aides have been using the lift machine that has a cradle, similar to a hammock. Three aides found the correct machine and brought it into the room. They proceeded to get Bob ready for bed by removing his shirt so they could put his nightshirt on him, which he objected to strongly. The Stranger is always nearby and trying to make trouble through Bob's mind and body.

One of the aides asked me to leave the room, which I did. After a short period, the nurse and two of the aides came out and said all was OK with my husband. The aide proceeded to tell me this chair lift is not the safest lift to use. The safest one is the type that you stand on, which was the one which Bob was on when he passed out and almost choked to death, when his legs gave way and the strap that holds the patient, slipped up to his throat. This happened on the 25 May 2007 when all of the same people were called to Bob's room. The nurses and aides were all the same except there was one different aide this time.

When the aide was telling me this long story, I remembered thinking this is completely opposite to what I was told 25 May 2007. I also remembered when Don and I were visiting, 11 June 2007, and the aide asked me if we had ever seen the hammock type of lift used before. I told her no we had not and she said she would show us how it worked. When she got Bob in bed, Don clapped his hands because it had gone so well and looked so easy to use. Also, Bob did not show any fear like he had shown when he was on the other type of lift and just before he passed out and started to turn purple and choke to death. One of the aides even remarked, when I told her that this machine frightened Bob, that most of the patients were frightened by it.

Sunday, 08 July

When I arrived at the Medical Center for my visit with Bob today, one of the aides called out to me that she had just finished feeding my husband. I do hope this is true because it gives me more "peace of mind" to know that Bob is still eating well.

When I returned to the Medical Center, about 5:30pm, a little later than usual, Bob was still sitting in his chair, in the reception room, which is next to the dining room. Two aides told me that they tried to awaken Bob to eat but they were not able to do so. I questioned several people to get a fresh plate of dinner for Bob. One of the kitchen staff told me she could do this. I asked her to get a small plate of spaghetti with meat sauce, which was on the menu for Sunday night, which she agreed to. She brought the plate with hot spaghetti, and it looked so good. Bob ate all of it except for one small spoonful. He also ate his usual ice cream sandwich.

Later when the aide brought his medication, she gave me the pills, which I put into Bob's mouth and he took some water and they were gone. This was so easy and I can't understand why they fool with the pudding and crushing the pills. I have asked them to put the pills in Bob's mouth for days, because it is so easy for him to take the medication this way, rather than mess with spitting the pudding out, etc…

Monday, 09 July

Today was very good for Bob. He ate well and looked especially clean and well-shaved. I see one of our favorite aides was on duty and she always does a nice job. This evening when I went back, after dinner, Bob was outside of the dining room still eating a piece of apple pie, which was great. The nurse gave him his medication by pill form, rather than mashing the pills and putting them into pudding, and it worked fine. Bob chewed up the pills, swallowed them and it was all over very quickly.

Later in the evening, I took Bob back to his room so I could wash up his legs and feet, arms and hands, and face, and put his nightshirt on him. It always seems to relax him some when I do this. It didn't work this time. When the two aides came with the lift, which was the hammock type, to put him into bed, he was like a mad man. His mouth was in a tight line and he was trying to hit anyone who got close to him with his fists, including me. When Bob saw the lift machine, it really set him off. I know the aides cannot lift all of the residents all of the time, but there must be another way that will work. I can only guess the Stranger took over when Bob saw the lift, which frightens him so much. The nurse gave him his medication and the aides decided to wait one hour, for Bob to calm down, before they tried again to put him to bed. He was still fighting mad when I left, which really hurts because I know this is the Stranger that has gotten into his mind and body.

Tuesday, 10 July

This day began like most with Bob clean, dressed, and

looking very good. I keep telling him that I wished he felt as good as he looks. While I was visiting with him the nurse practitioner came over to talk. It was a conversation that was interrupted with Bob, being very agitated, reaching for her clip board. She immediately went to get Bob an ice cream cone for him to eat and hopefully calm down. It didn't work as Bob ate the ice cream cone very quickly and continued to be very agitated.

At any rate, we finished our conversation, that was not very satisfying at this point. She did tell me that I was invited to be with Bob on Thursday when she and the Doctor make their rounds. I will be there about 11am.

I returned to visit Bob, after dinner, and was told he ate pretty good, which surprised me since he had the ice cream cone so close to dinner. I got there about ten minutes before 6pm and waited to see if Bob's medication would be given to him. Later, when Bob and I were sitting and talking he told me that he was sorry he lost his temper. He has said this to me before so I am sure, in my mind, he does know what is going on but he cannot control this Stranger when he is trying to take over Bob's body and mind.

Thursday, 12 July

The last few days have been about the same with Bob. No new information was learned from the meeting today, when Jim took my place as I had to go to the dentist. The meeting was with the nurse practitioner; the doctor was also supposed to be there but was not present. Jim was told roughly the same info that I was told yesterday, from the nurse practitioner.

They are still trying to adjust his medication. His medication will be given at scheduled times, as I requested several times. The staff will put a request in for elastic stockings, for Bob's legs to help reduce the swelling in his legs, which some of it is from the medication and some from his legs hanging down most of the day while he is confined to sit in the wheel-chair.

Bob is still having some good times in the early part of the day. Jim said he carried on a conversation with him for most of the hour visit. Jim also ate lunch with him and was surprised how well Bob ate and the amount of shrimp that he ate. It was mixed with pasta and some kind of sauce, and Bob really enjoyed all of his meal.

Bob asked for Barbe again today and if she were coming over tomorrow. I told him that she was planning on coming to see him for his birthday. I asked him if he missed her and he said yes, that it had been a long time since she was here. I told him that Barbe was here several weeks ago and that it was hard to judge the time. He said it seemed like a long time. I also told him that Don was to return from Hawaii on Saturday and would be over to see him as soon as he caught up on his rest after the long plane trip.

In the evenings, beginning about five thirty or a little before, the sundowning still takes over. The Stranger is there just as feisty as ever only now he has gotten a very loud voice. I asked Bob where he got that voice and he didn't know.

Bob is still very strong and fights for his life with anyone who gets close to him, including me, when this Stranger is working on him. This Stranger doesn't worry me as much as it used to because I know it is the Stranger making Bob so agitated and that Bob cannot control him.

I received a statement from Blue Cross & Blue Shield and one of the items listed was "Surgery" on 14 June 2007, and also a consultant had been called in. I am surprised that the doctor or nurse would not notify the family when something like this happens. They make sure the aide calls when Bob falls out of bed, at night, but no word when surgery is pre-formed. I will call Blue Cross & Blue Shield tomorrow and see what they have to say about this surgery.

Well I did call, and Blue Cross & Blue Shield told me that it was for some work that was done on Bob's fingernails. I called the Finance Dept. and they told me that it was for work that was done on Bob's toenails. I think the work was done on someone else. There is a man who resembles Bob very much and I think the work was done for him. Identification bracelets would help this problem.

Saturday, 14 July

Bob was a terror this am, but after I got over he calmed down a lot. He would not take his medication for the nurse but I was able to get him to take it. He had not eaten much lunch but that is OK as long as he eats one good meal a day. He took his 3pm medication very well. I asked the staff again to give him whole pills, not to crush the pills, and I was able to put them in his mouth, as he chewed them, and it was over without Bob spitting the medicine out of his mouth.

I went over a little before 5pm and Bob had eaten almost nothing, not even his soup. I took him back into the dining room, got him a bowl of soup that had been put into the blender and he loved it. He even dipped his roll into it and ate it all. I then got him a plate of hot mashed potatoes with thin slices of roast beef, onions, etc. He ate all of the potatoes, and some of the beef. I got another roll and made him a sandwich with the beef that was left, and he really went to town eating it. I think he really enjoyed it. Then he finished off with the inside of lemon meringue pie. We never did eat the crust. Then after he took his six o'clock medication, pill form, I got him an ice cream cone which I know he enjoyed.

It was a very good evening. I took him to his room, where it was quieter, and we watched Antique Roadshow. I got plenty of hugs and kisses and he was so like his old self.

Tonight I went back at ten o'clock to pick up his laundry and take over his blue sweater that he asked for, and to bring the white one home to wash, and found him sound asleep in bed. I was over and back in fifteen minutes by the shuttle, which is so convenient. The driver said she would have waited for me but I told her I wasn't sure Bob would be asleep in bed or I would have asked her to wait. What wonderful service! Naturally I would not awaken him from sleeping but it does give me "peace of mind" to know that he is in bed and asleep. Now I am going to enjoy my wine and go to bed.

Sunday, 15 July

Well today was uneventful. Bob did not eat breakfast, very early, which is rather normal, ate a big lunch, and even ate two bowls of strawberries, which is very unusual. He always gave me the strawberries.

When the nurse came over to give Bob his six o'clock medication, he took it and spit it all out. I asked her to bring the pills, which she did, and then I had no trouble getting him to take them. This is what helped calm him today, I am sure. He would sleep some and be alert some of the time today. Those crushed pills in pudding really leave a lot to be desired. It must be very sweet, as Bob says.

This evening I went back at four-twenty and Bob was still sitting outside where I had left him. I took Bob into the dining room and he ate very little, some of a chicken breast, which was very good, a small bowl of soup and a glass of milk. He did not want his ice cream so I let it go at that. Later on, I asked him if he wanted the ice cream but he still said no. He then slept from six-thirty until nine-thirty when the aide came in to put him to bed. The aide said I will have to take his shirt off first. So, Bob reached up and pulled his shirt off by himself. Bob wanted to stand. So I said to the aide, let's get on each side of Bob, and let him try. We moved the chair nearer to the bed and each took an arm and Bob stood, very shaky, but he stood long enough for us to turn him around and sit him on the side of the bed. It was so much easier on him and the aide. He did most of the work. I did not feel any weight from him. I thanked him for being on his good behavior, kissed him goodnight, and told him I would see him tomorrow; and he said goodnight and OK. I know he wanted to get back to sleep. This was one of the best nights for him and I hope he has a really good night because he went to bed without fighting the aides or the world. This was a very long day but I would not have wanted to miss it for anything. I am so glad I was a witness to him standing. Another aide has been telling me that she handles Bob like this in the morning and I really wondered how she could manage. However, after you use this method once, you do believe it will work. The night aide was very surprised also.

Monday, 16 July

Today was pretty good for Bob. Jim and I had a nice visit with him and when we left, shortly before his dinner time, he was still in a good mood. I returned to visit with Bob, after my dinner, and got over there a little before 5pm with our son, Don. There was Bob sitting, in his wheelchair, in the very same place his brother and I left him. The aides called to me, in unison, that he was acting up so they brought him out of the dining room The woman next to him was continually shouting and hollering and did not stop. The aide was trying to feed Bob and he was resisting. He did not seem agitated, to us, at this time. He just didn't want to eat. He has always become upset with loud noise of this type. He had eaten his soup and a couple of spoonfuls of the food on his plate and that was all he wanted.

Don and I took Bob back to his room for a visit, and in a short while I got him an ice cream cone which he ate like he was starving. I said to Don that he appeared to be really hungry. I keep telling myself that this is probably one of the better

124

nursing homes in the area. However, for a fee of over eight thousand dollars a month, the expenses are growing. Yes, that is correct, eight thousand dollars a month. I do not want to eat with Bob every night because I think he will depend on me too much and not work with the nurses and aides.

At six o'clock, I requested that his medication be given to him and in pill form. I noticed there was a new nurse on duty, who brought the medication to Bob's room after telling me that the order called for the medication to be given smashed and in pudding, etc. I guess another nurse told him this was OK, rather than have Bob spit the medication out of his mouth. Bob took the pills easily for the nurse and opened his mouth wide to show him that the pills had been swallowed. The pills work so much easier. The nurse told me later that Bob had taken his last pill of the day for him very easily which I appreciated because I know how important it is for him to have his medication. These little comments from the nurses or aides go a long way in giving me "peace of mind."

I left about seven o'clock and returned at eight o'clock and Bob was still asleep. He had taken his medication very easily, in pill form, when Don and I were visiting. At nine thirty, the aide told me that she would try and get him into bed. I told her the good luck we had the night before, when Bob stood for a few seconds, which was enough to help him sit on the bed and the aide lifted his feet up onto the bed. She agreed that we would try this method again, which we did, and it worked out okay. Bob did not stand as well as the night before but there was enough time to help him onto the bed, and the aide lifted his legs and swung them onto the bed as the aide had done the previous night. She worked quickly and finished up with Bob. I sat with him, in the dark, and he drifted off to sleep very quickly as he still had the medication in his system. One of the day aides has been telling me that she uses this method to get Bob out of bed in the morning and has had very good luck with it, rather than use the lift which frightens him so much. I am so glad she told me this because I do not think I would have suggested it otherwise.

Tuesday, 17 July

Things have changed a bit for Bob today. One of our favorite aides was back after having the weekend off. She came in and got Bob to change his protection brief. Naturally, he didn't like it at all, but he was so much more comfortable when he returned.

The situation was better at dinner time. I stayed over to make sure Bob was taken into the dining room, by me, and given a chance to eat. The lady who yells all of the time was moved out of the reception area while the meals were being served. Bob was only given medication pills today, which he took very well. I took him into the dining room and he ate his soup, most of a salad, all of his entrée—which was shrimp and scallops in a sauce with rice, and all of his mashed potatoes. He had Boston cream pie for dessert and I think he did very well. I was glad I was there to see all of this. I just came home, at seven o'clock, and have my dinner heating up now. I will go back about eight-thirty tonight for the last chores and to pick up his laundry.

When I went back at eight-thirty this evening, the aide who takes care of Bob gave me the signal to be very quiet as Bob was in bed and sound asleep. Therefore I was unable to do my chores, which I feel help relax Bob, so I will do them earlier tomorrow evening just in case he is put to bed earlier. This aide is very good and always uses the protection cream in the private areas to keep Bob's skin free of any rash. I mentioned to her that I had not seen the beeper on the pad on the floor, and she ran right back to his room as I left. This beeper sounds off if Bob falls or gets out of bed, which is good security. The aide also told me that Bob stood for her to get him into bed and it was not necessary to use the lift, for which I am glad.

I hope I didn't hurt Jim's feelings when I told him that I got "carry-out" for my dinner tonight instead of going to the dining room with him. He had made plans for us to go to dinner with two of his friends. I know he is trying to help me not feel alone, and to relax at dinner time instead of running back and forth. I still do not think it is a good idea to eat with Bob every night.

Wednesday, 18 July

The Nursing Home experience is really something you will never forget. I keep telling myself this is one of the best nursing homes I have ever been in. I went over to visit Bob yesterday, got there about twelve-thirty, and Jim was there with him. He had been to a doctor and stopped in to see Bob on his way home, which was very good. Jim told me that Bob had been given his medication and started to spit it out, when he told Bob to open his mouth and take the medicine, which he did. Jim left shortly and I spent the rest of the day with Bob. Bob seemed very calm for the rest of the day, sleeping a little and even eating a piece of carrot cake, which was delicious, but it also probably took some of his appetite away.

I took Bob into the dining room for his dinner and got him a nice little salad to put some shrimp on, that I had taken to him, and got him chicken and mashed potatoes, etc... He didn't eat all of his dinner this time and I was reasonably sure he would not because he ate the cake.

We went into the recreation room to watch some television and just visit. He became moderately agitated and worked on getting out of his chair for hours. The nurse came over and gave him his six o'clock medicine, which he spit out, although we did keep most of it in his mouth. Usually he will sleep for a couple of hours after taking his medicine, but not this time. I left at eight o'clock and he was still working hard to get out of the chair, which has a tray in front of him to keep him from getting out or falling out of the chair.

Bob spit out his eight o'clock medicine so the nurse gave it to him again in liquid form and put it in the side of his mouth. Bob continued to work on his chair and when I returned at nine o'clock he was still agitated. I took him to his room and did the wash-up chores, put his nightshirt on him, etc., which usually relaxes him and it did seem to. The medicine was also taking effect and he was getting sleepy.

His night aide came in at ten minutes to ten and we stood Bob up at the bed, turned him around and sat him on the side of the bed, and we each lifted up one leg and got him safely on the bed. The aide worked quickly and did a nice job of finishing up washing Bob, and covered him up and he looked so peaceful finally. I do hope he sleeps through the night. The aide told me that if he goes to sleep he usually sleeps through the night.

Many times when another aide takes care of him he either rolls out of bed or gets out of bed. I believe when he is so agitated, for hours, he is exhausted and will probably sleep through the night. This Stranger is awful and will not give up. He is determined to take control of Bob's mind and body.

Today another day aide changed Bob's protection briefs for the second day in a row. This was about 2pm. I can't figure out what changed the routine. I think the aide needed two other aides to help her. I know Bob doesn't like this but it is so necessary when he sits in this chair from about 11am until bedtime, which can be as early as 8pm or as late as 10pm, and that is a long time.

Thursday, 19 July

What a surprise I had when I went over to the Medical Center to visit with Bob today. I had a rather large bundle of clean clothes so I took them to his room, as I usually do, and planned on putting them away when I wheeled Bob down to his room later. There in his bed was a man, who strongly resembles Bob, sound asleep in his bed.

I went immediately to the front and ran into a man who asked me if I needed help. I told him my problem, pointed to my husband who was in his wheelchair at the nurse's station and inquired what next? He asked me to show him the room and we went down and he finally got the intruder to tell him his name and the intruder fussed as he didn't want to be awakened.

This man, whom I met at the front desk, happened to be second in charge of the whole Medical Center and he finally got the intruder to stand and turn around and sit back in his wheelchair, which was by the side of the bed. He even had his shoes on the clean sheets. Later they stripped the bed and the lady who straightens the rooms even wiped down the mattress and replaced all of the bed linens with clean sheets, etc.

For a third day in a row, the day aide changed the protection briefs on Bob. I don't know if she will be the only aide who does this or not. As I have said before, this has not been done since the first month Bob went into the Medical Center. Bob was on a light diet today as he did not feel good. One of the night aides and I got him into bed about nine tonight after I did my wash up chores and put the nightshirt on Bob, and he looked so peaceful and content in bed. I do hope he sleeps through the night and maybe he will feel better tomorrow.

Saturday, 21 July

Today when I arrived over at the Medical Center, 12:10pm, Bob was in his extended wheelchair in the hall at the Nurse's station, without going in to have lunch, which is from 10am until 12noon. I immediately took him into the dining room, opened the cabinet drawer and took a bib out for him, got him some juice and a platter of food. One of the servers, who works in the kitchen, fixed him the best looking hot turkey sandwich, mashed potatoes, and peas, which he really enjoyed. I gave him one spoonful and he took his fork from the table, and finished eating every bit of food himself. He really did a good job. Later, when he was supposed to get his medication, I got him an ice cream cone, which had nuts on top, asked the nurse to push his medicine into the ice cream on top, and I gave it to him. He certainly does like his ice cream and this was such an easy one for him to take his medicine. He slept most of the afternoon so I left after asking the nurse not to awaken Bob to take his three o'clock pill. The nurse told me this pill was for the pain Bob sometimes gets in his legs. We both wondered why he would get this pill at three and another of the same thing with his six o'clock pills. The nurse did not awaken him and said she would leave a note for the nurse practitioner and question this procedure. When I returned with Jim at 4pm, Bob was still asleep and did not know I was gone.

We took him into the dining room for his evening meal and started with one cup full of pea soup, with ham in it, which he enjoyed very much. I then got him another full cup and he enjoyed that one also. I then got him a nice little salad and that was enough for him, so we took him out of the dining room. As we were getting ready to move Bob out of the dining room, Jim leaned over to help lift Bob's foot back onto the foot rest and he noticed that Bob's pants were almost all the way off and soaking wet. No, he had not been changed all day, and in fact, the pants Bob had on were the same he had worn the day before. I requested two aides to change him completely, and since it was still dinner time they told me it would be a short while before anyone could help Bob. I said okay, and Jim and I took Bob back to his room where I removed his shirt, which was an outside jacket which the aide had put on him earlier. He had three complete outfits in his drawers, but Bob may have said he was cold and requested additional clothing. In a short while two aides did come and tended to changing all of the wet clothing. He looked very nice when they finished.

Later, at five forty-five, when the nurse came over with his six o'clock medicine, which is about six pills of various sizes, I ran to get the ice cream cone from the freezer, put all of the pills into the top of the ice cream and gave it to Bob. He ate it like he enjoyed it very much. This is so much easier than having Bob spit his medicine out of his mouth.

Bob slept most of the evening and it is no wonder he doesn't sleep at night. We will see what happens later and I do hope they put him to bed, although I know the staff is concerned if Bob goes to bed early, in a couple of hours he will be awake and out of bed. He was still sleeping in the chair at nine o'clock when I took his laundry and left to return home and do the wash.

Sunday, 22 July

The nurses are giving Bob two strong doses of Seroquel every day; it is used as an antipsychotic medication. I was over there, taking laundry at 8:45am this morning, and Bob was still sound asleep in his bed. In fact, it looked like he had not moved the entire night. He had his first medication at 10am, and it knocked him out for five hours, until 3pm. Even then he was not fully awake. The nurse said he was starting to get agitated! He was probably hungry and may even have had a change in his blood sugar. I do try and give him water or something to drink when he is awake. He had no breakfast or lunch, nothing to eat or drink since four o'clock on Saturday. He did have an ice cream cone about an hour later on Saturday, but nothing to drink until four o'clock dinner time today, Sunday.

He was so knocked out that I had the nurse check his vitals. His blood pressure was very low, naturally, since the Seroquel also lowers blood pressure. Its side effects cause the same symptoms as Parkinson's disease for which they are giving him Sinemet three times a day of two pills each time. When Bob was home he was taking one pill six times a day. I believe this increase could be too strong for Bob. The nurses are giving him medication for his legs at 3pm and 6pm.

I understood the doctor, when he gave us the prescription, said to only use the second dose when needed. I am writing a letter to his doctor, not the nurse practitioner, to question his medication.

I will hand deliver the letter below to Bob's new doctor:

> I understand you are my husband's physician. He is Robert F. Awalt and is in the Medical Center, to refresh your memory. I would like to have the schedule for his medicines, what they are, and what they are for, especially the six or seven that you prescribed for him to take at six o'clock. Naturally, I assume you did because you are his physician. He is so highly medicated that I am appalled at the state he is in at this time. It was bad enough the first three weeks Bob was over at the Medical Center, but I realized the nurses were trying to get him adjusted to his new surroundings. I am sure this is still true; however his system can only take so much over-medication.
>
> I went over to the Medical Center this morning at eight forty-five to take some clean laundry and found my husband sound asleep in bed. He looked like he had not moved the entire time he was in bed. He was not given his first medication until 10am, according to

the nurse, as he was becoming agitated. Please keep in mind that he had had no medication for his Parkinson's disease since 6pm Saturday. He was not only hungry, but his blood sugar could be affected. He was in a deep sleep until three o'clock and then not fully awake. He had no breakfast, lunch, or anything to drink since he finished dinner on Saturday. He did have an ice cream cone about an hour after his dinner on Saturday. I really don't know how you expect to have good results with treating my husband, when there is a complete disregard for a schedule. It was my understanding that his Sinemet was supposed to start at eight o'clock regardless if he is sleeping or not. Why not wake him up, give him his medicine and maybe even some breakfast, and let him go back to sleep if he chooses.

I do not believe it is wise to use Seroquel and I ask you not to prescribe it for my husband. I realize that he needs to be sedated, to a certain extent, but there must be some other medicine that would be just as effective for a Parkinson's patient, without the same side effects, and does not knock him completely out for five hours or more.

Thank you for your attention in this matter. Please call me or answer by email. I find the email very convenient since I am over at the Medical Center frequently.

Sincerely, Jane Awalt

I also was pleasantly surprised when the aide, who was taking care of Bob today, asked to excuse Bob so she could change him That was very nice. He looked clean and more comfortable when she finished. She also gave him a very good shave with a razor. He did look good but he was sound asleep most of the day.

Monday, 23 July

I hand delivered the letter to the doctor's office, and have received no reply from her by either the telephone or by email. I didn't think I would but there was always a chance I guess. I had a long talk with the nurse practitioner and she will order the Seroquel to be reduced every three days so there will be no patient withdrawal from it. The Sinemet was not doubled, but the dose was ordered to be given at three times a day, rather than six times a day. Three other medications will be reduced at different times so it is not all done at once. This makes sense.

Bob's wheelchair leg and feet support pieces were found and placed back in his room where they were originally. One of the aides had borrowed them to put on the chair of someone who was roaming the halls, late Saturday night, so that person could sleep in the chair. I knew a resident could not have carried both of them at once because they were just too heavy for the average resident to handle. I now have the wheelchair home until, if ever, Bob needs it again.

A favorite aide was back and sure enough at 3pm she took Bob back to his room and checked him to see if he was wet or dry. She returned saying he was dry and no changes were necessary.

I had a long talk with the Director of the unit and she remarked that she could see I was filled with anger and needed to speak with her and the social worker. I was shocked and felt nothing could be further from the truth. I told her I had no one to be angry with and that I was frustrated about the medication Bob was getting, because there were so many of them and they were still knocking him out completely. I then gave Bob a small box of chocolate milk to drink and left to get my dinner at 4pm. I returned at 5pm to take Bob into the dining room for his dinner. All he ate was a small cup of soup. After trying to get him to eat with no luck for an hour, we gave up. At 6pm, I told the nurse I would try and get Bob to eat his ice cream cone with the pills on top. This is such an easy way for Bob to take his pills. After some coaxing he finally ate the cone and seemed to enjoy it. I gave him a ride in his chair for about twenty minutes and he went to sleep for one hour and a half when he awakened for a drink. I gave him some water and then he was wide awake. When I left him he was working on his chair trying to get out of it. I hope he sleeps through, but I doubt it tonight.

Tuesday, 24 July

It is now 10am and still no answer from Bob's doctor, and I am surprised. I keep being told she is new and I wonder if she is a new doctor, not just new on this job of taking care of the patients in the Medical Center. Bob's doctor, who moved to Florida, was very caring and responsive to my questions.

No, the doctor still has not responded to my letter at this date and I frankly do not expect her to, or she would have contacted me before this time.

Bob spent most of the afternoon sleeping but it was a nice natural sleep and not a sleep that looked like he was in a coma or close to going into a coma. I had lunch with Don, our son, and Jim, Bob's brother, and we then went over to visit with Bob. The personal care for Bob has certainly been above average. I am very grateful for this because Bob does look so good. It is too bad the doctor of a patient does not keep the family informed as to medications and progress of the patient or lack of progress of the patient. Nurses and aides should not be the ones to give the family or patient this necessary information. It should come directly from the doctor. The doctors should realize what anxious times these can be for the family of a patient in Long Term Care, especially the family of a patient who has Parkinson's disease and is fighting the Stranger who is trying to take over his mind and body.

I left to have dinner at five minutes before 4pm and returned at 5pm to help Bob with his dinner. When I told the nurse I was leaving and would return later, she asked me if I would be back in time to help give Bob his medicine. I said yes and I was back in plenty of time. First I got a tray with his dinner and took it and Bob to his room where he ate a fine dinner. It was much better than the night before when he ate only a cup of soup. Bob does not handle a lot of noise very well and he never did. I asked him to let me know when he wanted his ice cream cone and he said he would, and he did in about fifteen minutes. He said he didn't want to eat it too late in the evening. I went to the nurse and got the ice cream cone and she put the medicine in the top, where the nuts are, and I gave it to Bob. He really enjoyed his ice cream and this is so much easier than fighting him to take his medicine and/or not to spit the medicine out. The nurses all appreciate this help and thank me very sincerely. If something happened later on that I couldn't get over there to help them, I hope the routine will be established that Bob could continue taking his medicine like this. Once again he was sleeping when I left and I hope he had a good night.

Wednesday, 25 July

When I got over to the Medical Center to see Bob today it was about 12:10pm. There was no attempt to give Bob any medication so I assumed the nurses had already given it to him. He was asleep and continued to sleep, in his reclining chair, in the recreation room until one forty-five when I took him to his room. There he slept until the nurse came in at 3pm to give him his first medication of the day. Jim was also there when the nurse told me this.

Since she did not say he was acting up, I can only assume he was asleep all morning and once again they would not awaken him for any reason, much less give him medicine which was to begin at 8am. The nurse finally got the medicine into his mouth, which was in pudding, and which is also harder for Bob to take as the pudding must be very sweet.

When I was leaving to go to dinner at 3:50pm, I asked the day aide not to take my husband into the dining room for his dinner. Since he had his medication at 3pm, I thought he would be asleep for a couple of hours.

The aide told me, without me asking, that Bob had a good night last night and did not fall or get out of bed, which was good news. She asked me why I didn't ask earlier and told me I could have asked the nurse, who was working the day shift, I told her I was giving the nurses a break by not asking any questions and she laughed out loud.

This evening when I returned, at 5pm, Bob was awake and I got him a tray of dinner and took both to his room. He only ate a coffee cup full of soup, nothing more. In about a half hour I finally got him to eat his ice cream cone with his medication on top of the ice cream and he did eat it like he enjoyed it very much. The nurse gave me the last half pill to give Bob at eight o'clock, which I did, and I had some ice cold lemonade for him to drink, which he did, and I then left.

As I was leaving the two nurses told me repeatedly how much they appreciated my help for my husband and for them. They hugged me, thanked me, and went on and on what a big help I was to them and to Bob. The one nurse ran after me, as I left, and thanked me again and said I should receive all of the support possible because of the good job I was doing. I put some special cream on the sores on Bob's legs and ears, and the cuts on his legs are beginning to heal. I am so glad.

The nurses made me feel really good after all of the trouble I have had trying to get the medication straightened out. I continued to tell the nurses I am trying to help and give my husband the best care that is possible.

Thursday, 26 July

Today has been the best day that Bob has had in a long time. I went to the dentist this am and got over to the Care Center a little after noon. Bob was wide awake looking all around and very low key. I asked him if he wanted to play Bingo with the group and he said okay. Well! We played and he even called one number that he had, to my attention, when I was distracted. He also won a game and when he was showed the prize basket, to pick something out, he said no he would rather have candy. The activities director got the candy basket and he picked out a chocolate bar, small, took the wrapper off and ate it. He hasn't eaten chocolate for a long time.

The aide told me at lunch time that she offered to help him and he told her that he could feed himself, which he did: hot dog, baked beans, roll, sauerkraut, etc...

I left him at 4pm and returned at 5pm and I was told he had eaten macaroni and cheese and stewed tomatoes. Later he ate his ice cream cone, with the medicine on top. At 8pm he asked me for a blueberry yogurt which he ate and seemed to enjoy. I put the cream on his legs, the cuts are almost gone, turned out the lights, put soft music on the TV and waited for the aides to come in and put him to bed. I will be surprised if he doesn't sleep through the night. He had no naps all day.

When I told Bob I was leaving and would see him in the morning, he held out both arms to hug me and kissed me and told me that he wanted to go with me. He held me for the longest time like this and my heart was breaking for him. I wish I could bring him home, to our apartment, but I know I could not handle him when the Stranger is working so hard to have control over his mind and body.

The nurse practitioner called me early today to tell me they were cutting down on his Parkinson's medication to four a day. I had gently suggested that I thought to jump into the double strength was just too much for him. They had been giving him two pills, three times a day, making six pills. He had always taken six pills, one at a time, six times a day. I am hoping this change may be one that was needed to help him get some quality time and not be drugged all day and night.

Friday, 27 July

Bob did not have as good a day today as yesterday. He slept most of the day again but I was told he did eat lunch as the Director helped him to eat. Another person told me that he had not been up very long when I got there at eleven forty. It makes no difference, as Bob ate so well this evening, I find it hard to believe that he had eaten earlier. He had a very large portion of meat loaf, mashed potatoes, peas and carrots, a generous piece of chocolate pie and a carton of chocolate milk, which he requested.

About twenty minutes later he asked me for his ice cream cone, and we put his medication on top. Naturally he does not know his medication is there but he does chew it. So, he may really know it after all. I had a little trouble getting him to take his last medication tonight but he finally did take it.

I stayed with him until he looked like he was falling asleep and the aides took over. It is easier to leave him this way and not tell him good-bye, etc...

I find it so difficult to keep my composure when I see how red Bob's eyes are sometimes like he has been crying. I can hardly see to type this entry because the tears are flowing and I know in my heart there is nothing I can do for him except to pray for him, which I do night and day.

I do believe there are some changes that are being made to the schedules. I had a long talk with the social worker today when she approached me. The talk lasted more than one half hour and she told me I should never feel that I could not ask questions. The social worker, in talking with me, could tell how frustrated I was concerning the medications that were given to Bob.

When I left tonight I again asked the nurse to make sure the aides did not use the lift that you must stand on when they put Bob to bed. The aides tonight were different ones and I thought they may not know of the awful experience that Bob had on this machine when he was almost choked to death. I will never take it for granted that they know about this situation.

Saturday, 28 July

Today was about the same with Bob. I asked for his medication to be given according to the schedule and it was moved up to an earlier time. I arrived at the Medical Center at ten minutes after twelve and I suppose the twelve o'clock medicine was given because Bob was so sleepy. He was sitting in the hallway eating a chocolate chip cookie, which was half gone. We went into the recreation room but he did not want to play Bingo. Jim came over and was reading some jokes and Bob really got a kick out of them. He laughed and seemed to enjoy all of them.

Later when I returned from eating dinner, I got a tray and took it to Bob's room to help him eat his dinner. He liked the soup but did not want anything else. I had ordered one of his favorites, which was veal parmesan, but he was so sleepy it was difficult to help him eat. I finally cut a slice of the veal and put it into a dinner roll, as a sandwich, which he did eat. He did drink his milk and that was it. Later he did eat his ice cream cone after I told him the nurse said he could have it early because he didn't eat much dinner. He did eat the cone like he was still hungry but he wanted nothing later.

The nurse gave him his six o'clock medication, in the ice cream cone, and when I asked her what all of the pills were for she exclaimed that they were his medicine that were due. I asked her if she was giving him his Ativan, which was due to be given at eight o'clock and she said yes because she was leaving at seven-thirty. He was still asleep when I left at eight thirty when the aide was going to put him to bed.

Sunday, 29 July

Today was better for Bob. He was awake when I arrived at the Medical Center for my visit with him. Shortly after, he did fall asleep. The nurse told me she remembered our secret and had given Bob his ice cream cone, with his medicine on top, and he had really enjoyed it. This is such an easy way to take care of this rather than have Bob spit out his medicine and fight everyone who tries to give it to him. I don't understand why the professionals don't think of easier ways to accomplish some of their chores.

Bob had eaten a good breakfast and lunch which would certainly make him feel a little better. He looked good and, as I have said before, my major problem is not with his care, which is now above average for nursing homes, but with getting his medication adjusted correctly and having the nurses keep to a schedule. Once again, tonight the nurse combined his eight o'clock medicine with his six o'clock medicine. The nurse told me she was afraid she would have trouble getting Bob to take his eight o'clock medicine, especially if I was not there. The eight o'clock medicine is supposed to last Bob through the night.

I stayed over, at dinner time, to help Bob with his meal. I had gone to an early brunch so I was not concerned with my later meal. I could not believe how well Bob ate, which was everything. He ate his soup, salad, mashed potatoes, chicken, sauerkraut, drink and later his ice cream cone with his medicine pushed in the top of the ice cream. I was so surprised. He had a fairly good evening without sleeping. He had some mild agitation but it was not bad, and at times he would listen to me when I asked him to stop and to remember that he told me he wasn't going to lose his temper again. I hope he will have another good night. He has been sleeping through the nights lately and that is a good thing.

Monday, 30 July

This was the first day for a long time that Bob has not had the tray across his lap to keep him from falling or getting out of the chair. He looks good and is clean. The aide must not have put the protection brief on correctly because I noticed a puddle under his chair when I got there today. Apparently he had urinated and it had gone right through whatever he had on his body.

One of the aides told me Bob had not gone into the dining room to get anything to eat and it was a few minutes after noon. I took him into the dining room and one of the aides got him the nicest tray of food. There was soup, pizza, and two or three other tasty items. Bob did not want anything except the pizza, which he really enjoyed with his juice and milk.

We had a nice afternoon and Bob slept off and on but was very calm. Before I left at three forty-five, I filled out his menu for dinner and asked the aides to take him in to the dining room for dinner and to help him eat if necessary, as sometimes he will eat by himself. One of our favorite nurses was on duty tonight and I was told later she helped Bob with his dinner. He did not eat very well so she got him a ham and cheese sandwich which he did eat. This aide is going to make a wonderful RN.

It was good to see two of our favorite nurses back on duty. These two have passed their board exams to become Registered Nurses. One nurse has one more year to go before she can take her board exams and I hope she does well. One of the nurses gave Bob his medication on the ice cream cone before I returned from dinner. She remembered how Bob takes his medicine so easily when he is given it on an ice cream cone. She will make a good nurse as she has good observation skills, looks for different ways to make the patients more comfortable, and is a good worker. She also did not combine his eight o'clock and six o'clock medications. I hope Bob had a better night because he did get his medicine correctly.

Don came over and had dinner with me and Jim. We then went over to see his dad and we all had a nice visit. I also introduced Don to some of our favorite nurses and to Larry who comes to visit his mom every day. He is so good to her.

Tuesday, 31 July

Today was about the same for Bob. He ate his lunch very well on a tray in his room, and he was very late in having the aides help him get out of bed and dressed for the day. This was another day that he did not have his protective brief changed. Tonight at dinner he ate very poorly. I even had trouble getting him to eat his ice cream cone with his medicine on top. He did finally eat it but it wasn't easy.

At eight o'clock, Bob held my hand and arm very tightly and he told me later that he was afraid I was going to leave him. He kept the medicine in his mouth for a long time. He drank a small carton of chocolate milk and still one pill was there in his mouth. I hugged him, kissed him and gave him my hand after getting him some cold water. Finally all pills were gone. He almost fell asleep and the nurse said she would see the aides put him to bed. I told her that I hated to leave when he was awake because he always wanted to go with me. It is too sad for me to keep the tears away, which I do not want Bob to see. I find it so difficult to deal with the Stranger who wants to take over Bob's mind and body. I keep trying but I am afraid this Stranger is going to win.

Wednesday, 01 August

Today was pretty good for Bob. He was still eating in the dining room when I arrived over at the Medical Center for a visit with him. He had eaten three quarters of a delicious sandwich and even had strawberry ice cream, I was told. I took him back to the recreation room and as I left with him I picked up a blueberry yogurt and a small box of chocolate milk. When we got over there Bob took the yogurt, opened it, took the white plastic spoon and ate it all by himself. I couldn't believe it and I wondered how satisfied he had been with his lunch.

When I returned after dinner to help Bob with his dinner, he didn't seem too interested in eating. He did eat his mashed potatoes and fish, which really looked good. I had a little trouble getting Bob to eat his ice cream cone after his dinner. I did wonder if he is getting wise to the fact that his medicine is on top of the ice cream since he chews the pills and swallows them without difficulty. We will be able to tell in the near future.

Later in the evening the nurse asked me if Bob had been given his noon medication when I was present. I said no medicine had been given to him while I was with him. I also told her that I had not asked the nurses, at noon, because sometimes they give Bob his medicine a little before the hour. I told her that he had a pretty good day in spite of not having the medicine. He slept a little, not much, was not very agitated, just a little, and seemed in a very good mood.

I did have some trouble helping the nurse give Bob his last medicine of the day, which was eight o'clock, before I left for the night. Finally, I got him to take the two pills and swallow them, but it took a long time before he got rid of them completely. I do hope he has a good night sleeping.

Thursday, 02 August

Most of today, Bob spent sleeping. I went over early to take laundry as I was not sure Bob had enough pants for the day, which it turned out he did. However, there he was in his chair, spic and span, having had a shower and all nice and clean but sound asleep. I put the clothes in his room and left to go to the dentist. I was back in less than one hour and the Director told me she had tried to feed him but he would have no part of it. I think he had been given his medication and he was in a deep sleep, which I saw. I got him a nice turkey sandwich, which he would not eat. Later on I gave him a container of blueberry yogurt and he drank a small box of chocolate milk. I asked the nurse to tell the aides not to take Bob into the dining room to eat because he had the yogurt so late in the day. I did not think he would eat any dinner. When I returned there was Bob in the dining room, he had eaten all of his dinner and was eating an ice cream sandwich. They told me he had eaten by himself, which was good. Each day is so different that it is difficult to guess what is going to happen next.

Friday, 03 August

When I went over to the Medical Center to visit with Bob today I received a great shock. It is just that when I think I have heard or seen everything and there can be no more surprises, another one happens. It was twelve forty-five and I didn't see Bob anywhere so I went to his room. There he was sitting on the side of his bed, still in his night clothes, and he had missed his breakfast and lunch. His security alarm was ringing with no one paying any attention to it. The nurse took it and put new batteries in it and said the aides could not hear the alarm when it went off. I am so glad he did not attempt to walk. It was like he was not interested in walking at all.

He had not had any of the medication that he was scheduled to have beginning at eight o'clock. I asked the aide for some cream chipped beef, which I know he likes, and she had already fixed him a nice ham and cheese sandwich, with a glass of orange juice, and a cup of apple sauce. He ate the cream chipped beef over two biscuits, orange juice, half of the ham and cheese sandwich and part of the apple sauce. He was really hungry and I am thankful that I could get him something that he really likes to eat.

I returned after dinner, about five-thirty and Bob was still sound asleep. Since no one approached us to give Bob any medicine at six o'clock, I assumed it was late because the earlier medicine had been two hours late. At eight o'clock I asked the nurse if she could give Bob his six o'clock medicine, which she agreed to. He was awake when I left him at eight-fifteen and returned home. I started to think that I better go back and stay with Bob until they decided to put him to bed. Well, I am glad I did go back. When I saw Bob sound asleep in the chair he was half falling out of it and looked very uncomfortable. I took him to his room and I asked the nurses to help him. Four of the aides and one nurse did help him get cleaned up, changed his protection brief and make him clean and comfortable for the night. Bob quickly went to sleep and I took his laundry and went home.

I do not understand how medical staff can have a schedule for medications to be given out and pay no attention to it at all. I believe it is like my brother-in-law Jim said that there is no recovery of the patients in long term care in nursing homes, so no thought is given to the scheduling and administration of medicines. The staff has one hour in which to give out the medicines to the patients. This delay may not effect some of the patients with their medicines. However, it does affect Parkinson's disease patients greatly, especially if the patient has reached the "down time". The patient then has a very uncomfortable time for a half hour or more waiting for the medicine to "kick-in" to help.

146

Saturday, 04 August

I arrived at the Medical Center about noon to find Bob very sleepy and guessed that he had been given his medication. He was trying to eat his sandwich, which he finally finished, and he drank two glasses of juice. I tried to keep him awake by putting cold and wet napkins on his forehead with little success.

He was clean and shaved and looked good. I asked the nurse if he could skip all of his medication except his Parkinson's medication, Sinemet, since he was so sleepy and far from being agitated. She agreed and I put the Sinemet in his mouth at twelve-thirty, thinking it would melt. Bob did awaken long enough to chew the pill and swallow it and then eat an ice cream cone, which was a good thing.

I checked his room and his bed was made up and the room looked fresh and very tidy. I also noted that Bob had on his support stockings for the second day. I washed them out last night and hung them on a towel bar, in his powder room, to dry. One of our favorite aides said she would order another pair of the support stockings for him to have in his room.

I finally found out the connection with the staff and the resident who screams and hollers so much. I often wondered why the staff did not sedate her so she would not upset the other residents. It seems her daughter is good friends with one of the nurses, and the daughter is an employee in the corporate offices. You live and learn when you are a frequent visitor. You can learn a lot about the care of your loved one and also what else goes on in the nursing homes especially when the staff thinks you are reading and not paying attention. I have never complained about what I see going on with others.

I also thought it was interesting that the nurse went around checking all of the security alarm boxes to see how loud they were. I wondered if this had any thing to do with Bob's situation yesterday, when no one answered when his alarm was

147

sounding when I arrived for my visit with him. The nurse changed the batteries yesterday in his alarm box, which is attached to Bob's chair and to him. The alarm is now very loud on his box.

Jim and I stayed over to eat dinner with Bob tonight. He ate his salad and went right back to sleep. He has continued to sleep this entire day. We finished eating and I made a sandwich for Bob with his crab cake in a roll, and we took Bob back to his room as he was still sound asleep. Finally he did awaken long enough for me to help him eat his sandwich and drink a box of chocolate milk. He immediately went back to sleeping, which doesn't seem normal. We can't figure out why they do not give Bob something to sleep at night so he can be awake at least part of the day. I stayed with Bob until eight-fifteen when he awakened and was wide awake, like he should be in the daytime. I took him over to the nurse's station and left for the night. I am sure he will not sleep much tonight after sleeping most of the day. Something seems wrong with this routine.

Sunday, 05 August

I arrived to visit with Bob about noon and he was dressed and in the dining room just finishing his lunch, which he had eaten very well. I was told he had been given his medication, which I believed because he slept all afternoon.

Two aides took Bob down to his room to change his protection brief at 2:30pm. I have the feeling that he was not even put to bed last night. He still had on his support stockings, which were inside out, and this was easy to tell because the Awalt name is on the stockings in very large print. Jim was over this am, shortly after 9am, to give Bob Holy Communion and found him in the wheel chair at the nurse's station. He said he had on his pajamas, which he hadn't worn since the first week at the Medical Center. He still had on his street

148

clothes with the pants legs pushed up to the knees, where I had left them after putting cream on his legs to clear up some small cuts that were there. Later his pants, from yesterday, were hanging in the bathroom on a towel bar to dry out. They were still very wet when I put them in the plastic bag to bring home. I guess they had not changed his protection briefs all night and day until they got him dressed, knowing that I was coming over for my visit with Bob. If the pants had been hanging there all night they would have dried by morning and certainly by the afternoon of the next day.

Bob ate very poorly this evening and now I know why. When I left I mentioned to the nurse that I thought Bob was unusually warm. She just called me on the telephone to tell me that he had a temperature of 102.4 degrees. She also noticed blood in his urine, which leads me to believe he may have a urinary tract infection, and the nurse agreed. I do hope he is comfortable tonight. I will go over early tomorrow.

Monday, 06 August

Bob has certainly taken a turn for the worse. He definitely has an infection in the urinary tract and has been started on strong antibiotics as of this morning. The Director and the social worker approached me when I returned from dinner and asked me how I felt about Bob's care if they couldn't get food or liquids into him. I told them he did not want any tubes, hoses, etc. or any artificial means of this type including IV for feeding. We had both decided this many years ago and I want the same thing to die naturally without prolonging the process artificially.

Don sat with Bob and me today, after lunch, for almost two hours and Bob did not respond at all. He continued to sleep this evening when I returned after dinner, 5pm until 9pm without responding at all. I held his hand the entire time and I could feel him hold my hand very tightly and then relax it somewhat and then tighten his grip again. I felt very surely that he knew I was there with him. I spoke to him some and kissed him without any verbal response. The nurse told me that they expect the antibiotic to help him within 48 hours, or else the infection will travel throughout his body. I guess once it gets into the blood stream that is how it travels throughout the body.

One thing for sure, he will probably sleep through the night, and not be able to get out of bed.

Tuesday, 07 August

Bob was sleeping most of the day today. He has certainly received good attention, if these prove to be his last days. I was able to give him a cup of ice cream, which he asked for, and some cranberry juice. He looks peaceful and clean and comfortable. It appears the Stranger is no longer trying to control Bob's mind and body. The many medications that Bob is given probably help to control this situation.

Wednesday, 08 August

Early today the new doctor was in to see Bob. She asked him if he was in any pain and he answered her that he was not. She asked him a couple of additional questions and he answered her. This information was given to me by the nurse practitioner. Naturally, I have not heard from the doctor nor did I receive any email messages from her. I think this is wrong. I believe the doctor should contact the family of a patient at least sometime. Apparently, this doctor doesn't agree that any contact is necessary with the family, even when it appears the patient is dying.

Bob was very poor today and that is why I just got home, 10:45pm, and I thought I would go back in a little while. However, I just received a telephone call from one of the nurses and she told me two nurses went in to check on Bob and he was wide awake. They gave him a cup of ice cream and he drank some cranberry juice and then he went back to sleep. I will probably not go back now, unless I receive another telephone call.

Thursday, 09 August

Bob is about the same today. He now has no more fight left in him. This is due to the strong antibiotic medication that he is now taking for the infection in his urinary tract; or he has just given up the fight. He sleeps most of the time and he is now in a recliner, with wheels, but has no tray across his lap, nor does it have any restraints of any type. He is eating very little and only takes a little water or cranberry juice from the end of a straw. He does not seem to have any difficulty in swallowing. I keep watching his feet and toes for any change in the coloring of his skin and toenails. The skin appears nice and pink and his nails have not changed in coloring. I sat with him until a little after 10pm tonight and I left with a very heavy heart.

Friday, 10 August

Bob has not changed much except he is very weak. He still is sleeping most of the time, and when his head is in my direction he looks straight at me but it appears he cannot focus his eyes. Yes, from time to time I still see a tear or two in his eyes. This really breaks my heart. I do not want him to see me crying but it is so difficult not to break down. I pray constantly to be able to turn off the tears but they just flow. As I sit here and type this Journal and think of him, the tears are rolling down my face. I will have to stop typing now.

Bob is still not eating very much. Today he ate a half cup of soup and drank a small container of milk. Later in the evening he did eat a cup of ice cream for me. I sit and pray for him for hours and I am very thankful he is in no pain. I am sure his pain is in his heart and mind. I know he knows I am with him because he will squeeze my hand once in awhile. One time he was able to raise his hand, while holding my hand, to his lips, as if to kiss it. I leaned over and kissed him and also kissed his hand. This is so difficult to do without crying. I expect and hope that the tears will dry up soon. The Stranger, who comes at sundown, is no longer a problem. Bob is too weak to be agitated.

Saturday, 11 August

Everything is about the same with Bob. When I went over to the Medical Center for my visit with Bob today, he was in the dining room with one of the aides feeding him. He looked so sad that I just broke down and cried. I could not help it. I turned my back, so he wouldn't see my tears and three or four of the staff came over to comfort me. I finally got my tears under control and took over trying to help Bob eat some food. He ate a little soup and a few spoonfuls of mashed potatoes. Later in the afternoon, I was able to give him a cup of ice cream and a small container of milk.

Bob looks very comfortable in the chaise lounge with wheels, and sleeps very well while he is in it. He is very weak and he has given up the fight now. He even opens his mouth to take his medicine without much resistance. He appears clean and dressed and also very sad. I stayed with him until the three aides and one nurse came in to put him to bed. I think he is too weak to get out of bed now. I kissed him good night and told him to try and remember I would see him in the morning. Once again, I left him with a very heavy heart. I am glad the final farewell has been said to the Stranger and I hope he no longer tries working on Bob's mind and body.

Sunday, 12 August

Today when I went over to the Medical Center to visit with

152

Bob I found him washed and dressed in the rolling chaise lounge. The aide told me he had eaten some food for lunch and also some fruit. I could not get him to eat tonight. All he ate was a half of a cup of soup and a small glass of cranberry juice. He only ate a half of a small ice cream cup later tonight. He rested with his eyes closed or slept most of the day. At one time I think he was watching a golf tournament which was on TV. He appears very weak but he can still give the nurses and aides a bad time when they get him ready for bed. He has always been so private, and now he can't get used to them washing him and changing the protections brief and generally making him comfortable for sleeping through the night. I do hope he has a good night. He seemed to understand when I kissed him good night and told him I would be over to see him in the morning. I just can't seem to take it when I see tears in his eyes. I feel so sorry for him that it is really painful for me to try and hold back the tears.

Monday, 13 August

Today I found Bob still sleeping most of the day. One of the very good aides had really gotten him washed and dressed and even used a regular razor to shave him. He looked so good. He did not eat much of his lunch as the aides told me. He ate about half of his soup, juice and half of his ice cream. Tonight when I returned after dinner, a wonderful LPN, who has just passed her Board exams, told me she tried to feed him and he didn't eat very much for her either. He ate a little soup, some fruit, and his medication which was in part of his ice cream, which he only ate half of that also. He did drink some cranberry juice and later I did help him drink almost all of a six ounce bottle of milk. He has some places all over his tongue and I thought maybe he has been drinking too much cranberry juice. The nurse said this condition may be caused by his Parkinson's disease. I also noticed there are dark red discoloring marks all over his feet. I do not know what this all means as I have heard nothing from Bob's doctor. I do not understand how a doctor can have a patient and have no contact at all with the family.

I left Bob after three nurses and aides got him into bed. I do believe he still has a little of the Stranger working on his mind and body but with little success. We were trying to get his shirt off while he was still in the chaise lounge, and he was holding his arms very tightly. I finally asked him to let me take his shirt off while the aide held him to prevent him from falling out of the chair. He agreed to this and relaxed his arms so I could pull his shirt off. I noticed all this time, while we were trying to remove the shirt, he had a big smile on his face. I thought the Stranger was gone because he seemed so weak. He still has a lot of strength in his hands and upper body but not in his legs.

I am going to try and find out what all of these places mean that are on his tongue and the feet. I guess the places on his feet could be associated with poor circulation. Maybe I can find out something on the internet to see if these red blotches are associated with the dying process since there is no contact from his doctor.

Tuesday, 14 August

Everything is about the same with Bob. He just won't eat and drinks very little. If you check on the internet, one thing they say is that this happens frequently in the last stages of Parkinson's disease. The patient just has no interest in eating or drinking. And, sometimes the body can't handle the food anymore. I helped him to have about four ounces of milk tonight. And, he ate a little of his ice cream, but not much. His face looked like it had a slight yellow cast to it. Jim suggested that his liver might be involved. His feet look dark but definitely not black, just dark. There is a faint sound coming from Bob's throat. It almost sounds like a very faint snore or even like a weak whistle. I am not sure what this sound might be unless there is fluid in his lungs. It almost sounds like there could be some slight congestion from his lungs.

Bob was more cooperative when the aides put him into bed. He put out his arms for me to take off his shirt and the two aides worked very quickly in washing him and getting him ready for bed for the night. He kissed me goodnight and when I looked at him, I thought how peaceful, calm, clean, and comfortable he looked. I do hope and pray that he has a good night.

Wednesday, 15 August

Bob was in the dining room when I arrived at the Medical Center today for our visit. He was adamant that he would eat nothing. He did drink three small glasses of juice but ate nothing. He only ate about one half a cup of ice cream which had his ground medication on top of it.

We went to the recreation room for a while and then to his room. He was sleeping most of the time and only occasionally opened his eyes. It is strange how so many times when Bob is sleeping, he smiles big and almost looks like he sees someone he recognizes. Jim was over, as usual, and we watched part of the ball game while Bob slept. At three o'clock I gave him a six ounce bottle of chocolate milk. At first I held the end of the straw and dropped small amounts of the milk into the side of his mouth. When he realized the milk was nice and cold and made his dry mouth feel good, he started to sip it with the straw in his mouth. It takes a long time to feed liquids into someone's mouth like this but on some occasions it is the only way to get liquids into a patient who is ill.

When the aide came into tonight to get Bob ready for bed I told her I would be glad to help her again. I think Bob is more comfortable when I help. At any rate, he was so funny tonight that we couldn't believe it was Bob. He made himself very stiff so that it was more difficult to handle him. All the while we were trying to get his shirt and pants off for me to bring home to wash; he had the biggest grin on his face. He finally tried to help a little with his feet on the floor before we turned him around to the bed. After the aide was finished washing him and putting the cream on him, he did look clean and comfortable. I laughed and told him that he won tonight and the aide was still laughing when she left the room. It is just amazing to me how much strength he still has in his arms and hands for not eating, losing a great deal of weight, and being so weak. At one point, he grabbed a hold of the aide's uniform and hung on to it very tightly. In fact, she had a time getting it away from him. He is something! That Stranger is not going to give up easily. The Stranger was probably celebrating tonight as he controlled Bob's mind and body once more and maybe for the last time, as I am sure the end is near for Bob to leave this earth and return to his Lord and Savior.

He was content in his bed when I kissed him goodnight and told him I would see him tomorrow. He gave me a kiss in return and I sat with him for a short while until he was asleep. I do hope he has a good night of sleep tonight.

Thursday, 16 August

Much is the same with Bob now. He is still not eating solid food and in fact today he would not take any liquids. Don came over to see his dad so we had dinner with him and Jim. It was a nice time and I did enjoy getting away for a short time. I think Bob knew Don was there to visit with him. Sometimes he looked like he was looking straight at Don or Jim or me. I have often thought he couldn't focus his eyes but now I am not so sure. He is still unable to speak or he doesn't because his voice is so soft and low. I continue to tell Bob he has his mother's soft and low voice that I cannot hear him

156

speak. I am so sorry I cannot understand what may be his last words. Some of his words are very low and some are garbled and neither Jim nor I can make them out.

Tonight I was able to feed Bob a small cup of ice cream. I took him back to his room at eight o'clock and washed his support stockings, so he would have them clean in the morning. I washed his legs and feet, hands and face, and his teeth. His gums look like they are starting to get a little red and I don't want him to have pain in his mouth. He has such good teeth and I hope he doesn't start to have problems with his gums.

I was able to get Bob's nightshirt on him and when the aide came in to wash him and put him into bed, she was very surprised to find he was almost ready. She worked very quickly and did a really nice job finishing up with Bob. He looked so peaceful and was ready to go to sleep immediately. This is the only time I have "peace of mind" when I leave him. I know he is clean and comfortable for the night. I am sure he will not be able to go on much longer without food or liquids. I am ready to give many prayers of thanks when it is all over for him. I am thankful that he has no pain. However, I do know how much he wanted to be at home with me. The only consolation I have is the knowledge that even though I am unable to finish caring for him, he is getting better than average care. I do what I can at the Medical Center for him but I know he needed professional help. The main problem I have had is the trouble the staff has had in trying to regulate his medication. That no longer seems to be a problem.

Saturday, 18 August

Today was much the same with Bob. He has still not eaten any solid food or taken any liquids. One of the nurses said to me today "You know what this means." I know she is trying to prepare me for the end, when Bob dies. I told her that yes, I did know, and I keep watching his toenails and feet to see if they start to discolor. I still cannot understand why I do not hear something from the doctor or nurse practitioner. It is only the aides or the LPN who give me any information if Bob eats or not.

I was able to get Bob's shirt off, to put in the wash, but Bob is dead weight now. He was unable to help with his arms at all. I told him I was sorry if I hurt him pulling off his shirt but I knew he would rather me do it than the aides. I would hug him and kiss him in between pulling off the shirt hoping it would distract him a little. It is so sad when I see a tear in his eyes. I don't let him see my tears but it gets harder and harder for me to turn them off so he doesn't see them.

I noticed the night nurse did put his medicine in his mouth, when I went to get a drink. When he was in bed, I noticed his Sinemet was still in his mouth but melting. I put some droplets of water in his mouth, which he swallowed and the Sinemet pill went down with the water. He was sound asleep when I left him tonight and I hope he has a good night. I am glad Bob has the "peace of mind" when he goes to sleep that he knows I am still sitting with him.

There were three new residents who came to the Medical Center. One lady was a neighbor of ours where we have our apartment. The husband is so sad. He reminded me of how I felt the first three weeks or so that Bob first went into the Medical Center. The other two are a married couple. The wife fell and hurt herself and the husband doesn't understand where he is or why. I guess the staff does get used to the changes of people dying and replacements coming in. It is all very sad.

Monday, 20 August

Nothing has changed in Bob's condition except he is not even taking a few drops of water or juice now. His eyes have been open for periods of time and these times he does seem to be able to focus them. I asked him if he could see me and he tried to answer yes. When Don was with him, Don asked him the same thing and Bob tried to answer yes. Bob still tries to raise his hand, while holding my hand, to his mouth, in an effort to kiss it, like he did previously, but now is unable to get his hand more than half way to his mouth. I just help him get it all of the way to his mouth and touch his mouth.

The aide came in to put him to bed at 8pm, and when she asked me if she could do so, I agreed. When I took off his support hose, to wash for the next day, I thought his large toe looked discolored; but it seemed to get a little better as the aide washed him and got him ready for the bed and night sleeping. I started to help her and she just picked up Bob by herself and placed him on his bed. I leaned over to lift his legs up and she lifted them up very quickly. He has lost so much weight that she had no problem in lifting him. He had his eyes open for a while and I kissed him repeatedly and told him I, too, would go to bed and see him in the morning. I stayed with him for an hour longer, after the aide finished up, and he was sound asleep when I left for the night. Bob is still washed and dressed everyday and looks clean and very comfortable in his big lounge chair. There is no fight left in him now but he certainly did try hard to be independent of all help taking care of him. Sometimes he has his hands closed in fists appearing to want to fight anyone who gets near him, but he is much too weak now to hurt anyone. The Stranger is no longer in Bob's body.

I asked the nurses, on different shifts, if they thought it was a good idea and could work out if I took Bob home to die. They are all of the same opinion that I should not do this. They indicated there may be a problem, if he was home, that would require medical help to relieve pain, but I would be unable to get this for him immediately and I too, would suffer with him. Also, they were all of the same opinion that he would not know the difference, at this point, whether he was home or in his room at the Medical Center. They also had some concerns for me that I would be with him almost 24/7 and would not take care of myself. Our daughter, Barbe, insists that I make the choice myself and do what I want for Bob. Don, our son, said it was out of the question because none of us knew what is yet to happen to Bob and the nurses and aides would be able to handle any surprise situation at the Medical Center. This is very good reasoning.

Tuesday, 21 August

I am glad I didn't move Bob back home to die. He is close to death now but still getting professional care. The nurses moved oxygen back into Bob's room, in case he needs it in his final hours. They also have orders ready to give him morphine as an aid to help his last breathing if he needs it. In some cases the breathing is so labored that the morphine can slow the breathing down and helps to keep the patient more comfortable. He is checked by the nurse or aide to make sure he is dry and comfortable. He is turned in his bed every two hours to also help him retain the comfort level.

Bob continues to squeeze my hand when he is not sleeping, which is most of the time. He has his eyes open at various times and then goes back to sleep. The nurse asked me if I wanted to have Hospice Service come in for the last days, which I declined. I have great support from family and friends and I personally think Bob is more satisfied with the quietness, in his room, without more people around. The Stranger is definitely gone from his body and it won't be long now that Bob has completely lost his battle, not only with the Parkinson's disease but the Stranger is at last defeated.

Saturday, 25 August

Bob died 24 August 2007, at 9:30am very peacefully. He

just slept away. Don and I were with him the night before he died and he looked clean, comfortable and extremely peaceful. Don mentioned he was glad to see him so peaceful, breathing easily but very quietly. He half opened his eyes a couple of times and appeared to look straight at us. Sometimes when he would open his eyes it seemed like he could not focus them. This time it looked like he could actually see us. I tried to keep speaking to Bob, as I was told the hearing is the last of the senses to go when someone is dying. I kept telling him that Barbe would be here the next day, thinking he could wait to say good-bye to her, in his own way, but it was not meant to be. She arrived Friday night and I was so glad to see her and have her support, with Don, Kathy, and Beth.

These last few days have been very quiet while sitting with Bob. Occasionally we would speak to him, sometimes he appeared to still hear us and other times he would be in a deep sleep, even snoring. The staff continued to keep him spotlessly clean and even shaving him.

The routine at the Medical Center in these last days was unbelievably caring and helpful. The last few days they would bring in a cart with a large bowl of fresh fruit, a basket of packaged snack foods, pretzels and chips, three large pitchers of cranberry juice, and orange juice and fresh ice water. There were lotions, pencils and pads, and generally anything that might be needed to jot down notes. The lady in charge of the activities even brought in the radio, tape and dvd player, with tapes and discs to play so we could have soft music. They were all so thoughtful coming in with hugs and kisses and offering many prayers, for both Bob and me, which I welcomed.

My thoughts, in retrospect, are that the staff needed to get to know me better and I certainly needed to know them better. The personal care given to Bob was outstanding in most cases. My major concern, in most cases, was getting the medication adjusted correctly. I could not understand why the dosage of medicine had to be so strong, at first, and then back off to a lesser amount. I understand the patient and the staff had to be protected from someone who at times was very combative. This was my problem and I do believe the staff had the experience that they knew exactly what they had to do. They also had the knowledge and experience to deal with Parkinson's disease and with "Sundowning" and the Stranger who took over Bob's mind and body. Many times when I asked Bob if the Stranger was in his body, he answered yes but there was nothing he could do to control him.

I still cannot understand how a doctor could examine a patient, or at least check his chart regularly to change medicine, increase the dosage or decrease the dosage, and generally make some changes and never have any contact with the family of the patient.

The excuse that a doctor might be new on the case is very weak. The doctor could call the family of the patient, telling them that he or she didn't know the patient very well but that would be corrected in time. The doctor could spend two or three minutes on the phone with the family member, and at least show some interest in the patient and his or her family. In my case, not knowing anything that was directly from the doctor treating my husband was one of the worse experiences I have ever had with doctors. Our former doctor understood that I could not always answer the telephone. I would email him questions or the result of trying a different medicine for Bob, and he would email me a reply almost immediately. Sometimes it would be two or three in the morning before I could get to the computer but I was always able to answer him before the next day. He was wonderful and gave me such "peace of mind".

My suggestions for any doctor, who may happen to read this Journal please have some contact with the family of any patient who is suffering, especially with Parkinson's disease. This disease can almost destroy entire families who might be trying to give some quality of life to the patient.

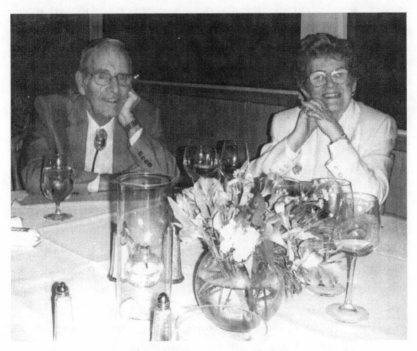

Bob and Jane Awalt

The Funeral and Its Preparations

Saturday, 25 August

The Funeral Director came to the apartment to go over all of the expenses for the funeral, and to pick up the clothes for Bob. I told the Funeral Director that both Bob and I decided a long time ago that we wanted to have the caskets closed. I will, however, check Bob to make sure everything was done properly and to see how he looks. Don and Beth are designing, and compiling the program for the funeral service which will be a Mass of Resurrection. Msgr. William J. Awalt will celebrate the Mass with Deacon James Awalt, John E. Awalt, and Don Awalt all taking part. Mary Margaret and Michael Cameron Farrell will present the gifts.

The pallbearers will be Don Awalt, Michael Cameron Farrell, Robb Farrell, Tim Edgar, James Manning, and Mark Metzbower. There will also be a Navy Honor Guard and they will play taps and present the American Flag to the widow at the cemetery when the service is over.

I knew expenses were going to be high but these are really astronomical. I do not see how the average family can afford to die. I realize that many people may have insurance policies to take care of this expense, but I wonder what the people do that can't afford to carry and pay for these policies. The shock of the Medical Center monthly fee, a little over eight thousand a month, depending on the number of days in the month, plus the fees for doctors and medications, was awesome.

I thought the fees might be a bit lower for the Funeral Home and the Cemetery but there was little difference. The expenses for the Funeral Home were a little over seven thousand and the prices for the services at the cemetery were also a little over six thousand. Most people that I have spoken to figure, as a rule of thumb, that you should allow roughly twenty thousand dollars for the complete funeral and I think the total will be close to this figure. I am so glad that we already have our burial site. The prices for grave sites now are staggering. Medical bills continue to arrive.

These figures do not include the casket, which was purchased previously from the Trappist Monks. Their caskets are all hand made and include many prayers while they are being made plus the fact that they are truly beautiful, especially for anyone who loves the natural wood. This casket will have a small cross carved into the top of the casket. It is truly beautiful as I saw when I first looked at them on the internet at the site of the Trappist Monks. This casket is also blessed prior to shipping and has a certificate included with the casket stating the date and all of the information. Delivery of the casket is promised for two days unless it is needed before that time and it did indeed arrive as promised. Arrangements can be made if delivery is needed before the two days.

Barbe, our daughter, and I made contact with the catering people to make arrangements for a light lunch, which will be after the funeral. It is very difficult to estimate how many to prepare for. We could only guess about one hundred will attend and hope these caterers will provide for more than that if necessary. I do hope there is enough food that they do not run out and disappoint anyone who attends. We allowed around one thousand dollars for this affair and it was a little over this amount. The caterers did an excellent job and they did not run out of food. The hall was very tastefully decorated with some flowers on the tables and the room looked lovely.

The Death Notice was in the paper and the wording was all correct. Many friends told me of errors in the paper when their loved ones died. The local newspaper reporter called today to secure additional information for an Obituary Notice to be in Monday's newspaper. The death notice will also be printed in Monday's newspaper. It is difficult to notify friends and relatives when a death occurs on a weekend. The reporter wrote an excellent Obituary Notice based on her conversation with me on the telephone.

I am amazed at the many cards and telephone calls from friends offering their best wishes, prayers, and condolences. It is very heart warming and I do appreciate their efforts very much. I have asked in lieu of flowers that memorials may be made to the Scholarship Fund, where we live, or The Johns Hopkins Parkinson's Disease and Movement Disorders Center in Baltimore, Maryland. Any and all proceeds from the sale of this book will also go to The Johns Hopkins Parkinson's Disease and Movement Disorders Center. It is my hope that with the publication of this Journal, someone who has Parkinson's disease or their family may receive some benefit from reading this Journal.

Tuesday, 28 August

It is now seven-thirty, the day of the Funeral for Bob, and Barbe and I are almost ready to leave for the Chapel here at the Retirement Home where Bob and I have lived for eight years. The visitation will be held prior to the Mass of Resurrection, which Bob's older brother, Rev. Msgr. William J. Awalt, will celebrate. Bob's other two brothers, John E. and James L. Awalt, will also take part, as will our son Donald, nephew Michael Cameron Farrell, and his wife Mary Margaret Farrell.

It appears to be a nice sunny day although it is supposed to be warm, in the eighties. Everything should be ready. There is one very large, beautiful flower arrangement, sent by our son and his family, and I was so grateful because it kept the Chapel from looking bare. They were lovely and this was a very thoughtful gesture from them.

The Mass went very smoothly and the singing was sad but very meaningful to me. The vocalist had a beautiful voice and the organist played perfectly, we had an early light luncheon, which followed the Mass, and then went to the Cemetery. The caterers did a super job on very short notice and I was very pleased with the results. The sandwiches and sheet cake that were left were sent to the Medical Center for the staff and residents to enjoy in memory of Bob.

I must say at this time, the turnout of friends, relatives, and acquaintances was outstanding. I could not imagine so many paying their last respects to the family in my wildest dreams. It was really overwhelming. The many cards and Mass cards are greatly appreciated.

The Interment at the Cemetery was very sad but tastefully handled. The Navy Honor Guard played Taps, folded the American Flag, and presented it to me. I will have the flag placed in a case to be hung on the wall in our apartment. Everyone at the Cemetery was caring to deal with. I will return to the Cemetery when the marker is in place and place some flowers on the grave site for Bob.

As I reflect and look back on the last three and one-half months Bob was over in the Medical Center, I have a warm feeling in my heart that the staff really work very hard in caring for the residents who are so ill. The residents have many problems that the staff has to work with. Many are there suffering with Parkinson's disease, dementia, and other serious illnesses. There is no recovery with these residents, yet the staff keeps their composure, never losing their tempers or their patience. I never heard any outbursts of anger like you read in the papers happening sometimes in Nursing Homes. The staff had much experience caring for people who had Parkinson's disease and especially the aides seemed to have so much dedication and compassion not only for the Residents but I was always included in their concern for my well being. I did not understand this feeling, at first, but it was soon apparent how genuine their compassion was for all concerned.

I began this Journal when there were many changes taking place in my husband's mind and body. My hope and prayer now is that anyone reading this Journal who has Parkinson's disease, or if someone in their family has this disease, they will learn they are not alone with these problems. I want them to also know that not all patients suffering with this disease have all of these same reactions and symptoms. This is a slow-moving disease and as different as we all are; so are the people who are suffering with this disease. Bob had this disease for more than fifteen years. Many do not have the disease for this long a period of time. He did well for a number of years but the last year was his hardest. The last eight months were terrible and the last eight days at home were so bad that I do not know how either one of us survived when Bob became very combative. It was apparent the Stranger had won and was clearly taking over Bob's mind and body. Bob always knew this as I continued to ask him if the Stranger was in his body and he always answered yes, but he couldn't do anything about it. He could not change the direction the Stranger was going.

We spoke with Bob's original doctors, the one at Johns Hopkins and the other who worked with the doctor from Johns Hopkins, many times about the different types of brain surgeries to correct this accident from Mother Nature. We were always told Bob's symptoms were not severe enough for brain surgery. There were also numerous studies testing new

168

medications that we kept trying to have Bob participate, without success. We were always given the same response that he had the disease too long. The studies required early diagnosed patients. Bob was fortunate, in the sense that even though he had taken Sinemet, the Parkinson medication, for more than fifteen years it still continued to help him. It is true it did not last in his body as long as previously, but it continued to help him some. This is not always the case with patients who have to take Sinemet for long periods of time. Bob had been spared some of the worse symptoms of the disease, which happen to some Parkinson's patients but not all.

At the end of this Journal I will list the websites that have much information about Parkinson's disease and they helped me considerably. I felt I could work with the problems connected with the disease better by learning more about it. I will also list some of the Support Groups that are available for not only the patients but the families of people suffering with Parkinson's disease.

Bob and I attended a Support Group for a number of years until he was unable to do so. The meetings were very informative with speakers who were physical therapists, speech therapists, vendors who sold helpful equipment for use in homes, patients who exchanged what happened to them and how they handled those situations, and they discussed the different medications. Sometimes a speaker would discuss some of the different medications that were being tested or coming on the market soon. They were interesting meetings and helpful.

I direct this last paragraph to any doctor who may be reading this Journal. In the last period of my husband's life, his personal doctor had no contact with me or any member of the family. The best information I found, when I was desperate to know if I was doing as much as possible for my husband, when he was in the last stages of Parkinson's disease, was on the internet. My thinking is this information should have come from the doctor to the patient's wife or family. The one bit of information I found to be helpful was the fact that near the end, the patient loses all interest in eating or drinking, and in many cases the body cannot handle the food so it makes little difference if the patient eats or not. I never tried to force Bob to eat or drink but I did spend a lot of time trying to encourage him to eat. When it appeared he might be having trouble swallowing I would put small amounts of liquid in his mouth by holding the end of a straw closed, to keep the liquid in the straw. I am sure if a doctor had spent just a little time with me I would not have worried so much if Bob was getting his medications on time or not. This situation can be very upsetting for the family of a Parkinson's patient and I believe it could have been helped tremendously by having some consideration and contact from the last doctor involved, either by telephone or in person. I visited with Bob at the Medical Center everyday and I believe there were many opportunities for the doctor to meet with me, either by telephone, email, or in person. All of the staff knew the times I would be available, so in my mind it would have been easy for an interested doctor to have contacted me or Bob's brother, who also visited with him every day.

All of the profits realized from the sale of this Journal will go to the Johns Hopkins Parkinson Disease and Movement Disorders Center in Baltimore, MD, (100 N. Charles Street, Baltimore, MD 21201) with the hope and prayer that a medication will prove to help stop the progression of the disease if not the cure of the disease. If anyone reading this Journal would like to contribute to The Johns Hopkins Parkinson's Disease and Movement Disorders Center, your monies would be most welcome; for this is what it will take to complete the research to be successful to help the many people who suffer with this disease. Contributions can also be made to the University of

170

Maryland Department of Neurology (University of Maryland School of Medicine, University of Maryland Medical Center, N4W46, 22 S. Greene Street, Baltimore, MD 21201).

I know how peaceful and content Bob looked when he closed his eyes and went to sleep. In my heart I will always be sorry I couldn't do more for him, but I was unable to help him when the Stranger had control of his mind and body.

A Parkinson's disease (PD) diagnosis can bring out so many difficult emotions—fear, anger, resentment, hopelessness, and more. It is a big challenge to learn how to cope with these feelings along with the stress of diagnosis and treatment.

Education and Support Groups can be an essential key to successfully coping with an illness like PD or other movement disorders. Studies show that the Information, training and counseling participants receive at support group meetings enhance quality of life, lower stress, and may even boost immune systems. (Courtesy of The Johns Hopkins Parkinson's Disease and Movement Disorders Center)

Things I Learned While Being a Caregiver for a Parkinson Patient

One thing I did learn (and I cannot emphasize enough) was the importance of exercise for the patient. Bob was so faithful, as long as he could, even when watching TV he would exercise his ankles, legs, and arms. This exercise helped him a lot. Many times Bob would use small hand weights to try and keep the muscles in his arms working so he could help himself in getting out of bed when he rolled over. He needed strong arms to help push himself up to a sitting position where I could then help him stand briefly to sit in the wheelchair.

Another thing I learned was to give Bob his medication as close to scheduled time as possible. This is why I complained so much at the Medical Center when they did not keep to a schedule. They had one hour which they could be off and it gave me a fit. With many medications, it may not make a difference, but with the Parkinson's medication it makes a big difference. The old saying "One ounce of prevention is worth a pound of cure" is true with most Parkinson patients. Once the "down time begins you have to wait for the medication to kick in and sometimes this can take a half hour or longer. During this time the patient is very uncomfortable.

I learned also to pray with intense feeling every day for strength and reasonable good health to continue as a caregiver, for patience to remember this is not my husband when the Stranger is in control of Bob's mind and body, and the ability to make the correct decisions in caring for Bob. As the months rolled by I prayed with more fervor and more frequently throughout the day. I believe much prayer is essential in surviving these trying times. My faith helped me tremendously.

I am very grateful to be settled in this retirement community and not have to make a move. I have had much love and friendship and fantastic support during this period of my life and will enjoy the many memories in my memory bank.

Things I Learned

- Keep to a schedule of giving medication so the "down time," when the medication wears off, would be kept to a rare happening. It is most important to follow directions daily.
- Keep to a schedule with personal care, i.e. shaving, bathing. Make sure there were no shortcuts and help them keep clean and fresh like they were used to when they were healthy. There should be no surprises if things were kept as normal as possible since most of us are creatures of habit.
- When your loved one can no longer hold a tooth brush easily, have them lie down on the bed so you can reach all their teeth and brush for them. You can also help them use a water pick so their gums and teeth will not cause them additional problems.
- Give comfort and confidence frequently, especially praise for small accomplishments or even for trying to attempt difficult tasks.
- When their legs hurt from the neuropathy, rub them with lots of massaging. Most of the time this routine really helps to relax them and they become more comfortable.

- When they are unable to use a walker (it is not hard to fall over a walker head first to the floor), it can be very helpful for them to walk behind a wheelchair pushing it. When they tire they can sit in the wheelchair and you can continue to push the chair.
- Exercise was very important and you can casually remind them to do their exercises even when they were sitting watching TV or listening to the programs.
- Hold the end of a straw to trap liquid inside and drop the liquid into their mouth when they are unable to drink or suck on a straw.
- Put bells on the front door and the door to their room so you can be alerted if they opened either door.
- Suggest crawling if it becomes impossible for them to walk, and eliminate the possibility of worse falls.
- Recognize that they may get upset if they are in a group of people. Strangers coming to help care for them may become out of the question. Just the thought of it can upset them. This may be one reason they may have a hard time accepting medical staff caring for them.
- Recognize how much they looked forward to being clean—washing their legs, feet, hands, arms and face each night. They may relax when you do these chores caring for them.
- Learn how much they like small things like ice cream. Even ice cream may help make it easier for them to take their medication pushed into it rather than fight them to take it. It may be much easier for them to take medication this way.
- Look for ways to prevent your loved one from becoming agitated as a daily routine.
- Secure easy access to a washer and dryer.
- Have back-up help if needed.
- Find a good care facility before you need it. Be aware that

you or someone else needs to go every day to let staff get to know you, watch the patient, and make sure the patient is cared for and not forgotten.

- Arrange your finances; it can take a lot of money to arrange for care and support.
- Remember the Stranger is not the patient.

10 Tips for Family Caregivers

- Take charge of your life—don't let your loved one's illness or disability always take center stage.
- Remember to be good to yourself. Maintain your own health through exercise, nutrition, and proper rest. Take time to do the things you enjoy and maintain contact friends and family.
- Watch out for signs of depression and don't delay in getting professional help when you need it.
- When people offer to help, accept the offer and suggest specific things they can do.
- Educate yourself about your loved one's condition. Information is empowering.
- There is a difference between caring and doing. Be open to technologies and ideas that promote your loved one's independence.
- Trust your instincts. Most of the time, they'll lead you in the right direction.
- Grieve for your losses and then allow yourself to dream new dreams.
- Stand up for your rights as a caregiver and a citizen.
- Seek support from other caregivers. Consider attending a support group or program for family caregivers. There is great strength in knowing you are not alone.

Adapted with permission from 10 Tips for Family Caregivers, National Family Caregivers Association.

Recommended Reading

Lucky Man: A Memoir by Michael J. Fox
Hyperion, 2002 ISBN 0-7868-6764-7

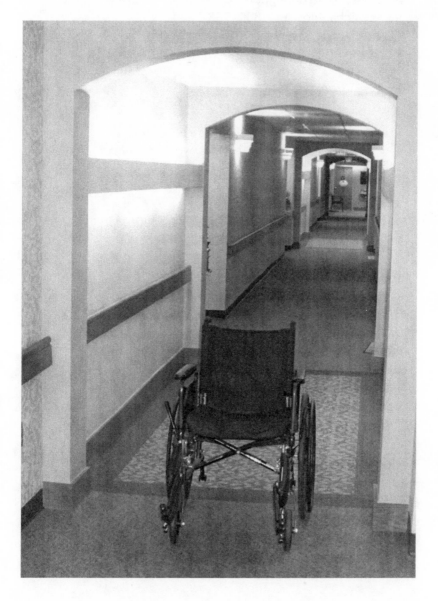

Parkinson's Disease Advocacy Organizations

American Parkinson Disease Association Inc.
www.apdaparkinson.org (800) 223-2732
1250 Hylan Blvd., Ste 4B, Staten Island, NY 10305-1946

Michael J. Fox Foundation for Parkinson's Research
www.michaeljfox.org (800) 708-7644
Grand Central Station
P.O. Box 4777, New York, NY 10163

National Parkinson Foundation, Inc.
www.parkinson.org (800) 327-4545
Bob Hope Parkinson Research Center
1501 N.W 9th Avenue Bob Hope Road
Miami, FL 33136-1494

The Parkinson Alliance
www.parkinsonalliance.org (800) 579-8440
P.O. Box 308, Kingston, NJ 08528-0308

Parkinson's Action Network
www.parkinsonsaction.org. (800) 850-4726
1000 Vermont Ave., NW Ste 1120, Washington, D.C. 20005

Parkinson's Disease Foundation
www.pdf.org (800) 457-6676
William Black Medical Building
Columbia- Presbyterian Medical Center
710 W 168th St., New York, NY 10032-9982

Parkinson's Disease Caregiver Information
www.myparkinsons.org

The Parkinson's Institute
www.thepi.org (800) 786-2958
675 Almanor Ave., Sunnyvale, CA 94085-2934

Professional Medical Associations

Movement Disorders Society
www. movementdisorders.org
(414) 276-2145
555 East Wells Street, Ste 1100, Milwaukee, WI 53202-3823

National Institute of Neurological Disorders and Stroke
www.ninds.nih.gov
(800) 352-9424
P.O. Box 5801, Bethesda, MD 20824

Parkinson Support Groups in Maryland

Allegany County Group

Call for information
Sharon Metz 301-689-3157

Anne Arundel County Group

4th Tuesday of the month, 12:00 noon
Elks Lodge in Severna Park
Truck House and Jennings Road, Severna Park, MD 21146
Ralph Luther 410/360-9480

Baltimore County Group

2nd Thursday on the month, 2pm
Johns Hopkins at Green Spring Station Pavilion II
        (Go through Cafe)
10753 Falls Rd., Lutherville, MD 21093
Becky Dunlop, RN 410/955-8795

Baltimore County/Charlestown Group

1st Thursday of the month, 10:00am
Charlestown Retirement Community
715 Maiden Choice Lane, Catonsville, MD 21228
Nicole Brandt 410-706-1491

Baltimore County/Oakcrest Support Group
3rd Thursday of the month, 1:30pm
8800 Walther Blvd., Parkville, MD 21234
Erica Reeves 410/882-3248 x 3218

Baltimore County/Kernan Group
2nd Tuesday of the month, 12:00 noon
Kernan Hospital
2200 Kernan Dr., Baltimore, MD 21207
Linda Miller 410/448-6867

Bethesda Carepartners Group
Chevy Chase Young Parkinson Network
3rd Thursday of the month, 7:30pm
The Carlton Condominium
4550 North Park Avenue, Chevy Chase, MD 20815
Leon Paparella 202-966-4450

Bowie Group
4th Monday of the month, 10:00am
Bowie Senior Center
13212 Oystercatcher Ln., Bowie, MD 20720
Ed Weisse 301/262-0947
Carter Rardon 301/412-0835

Carroll County Group
4th Tuesday on the month, 2:00pm
Westminster Senior Center Classroom
125 Stoner Ave., Westminster, MD 21157-5451
Marsha McMullin 410/848-2244

Chevy Chase Parkinson Network
3rd Thursday of the month, 7:30pm
The Carlton Condominium
4550 North Park Ave., Chevy Chase, MD 20815
Sue Hamburger 301/654-5572

180

Delmarva Group
Last Tuesday of the month, 1:30pm
Mallard Landing
512 Bluff Road, Salisbury, MD 21801
Milly and Wendall Daugherty 410-677-0333

Dundalk Group
3rd Monday of the month, 6:30pm
Ateaze Senior Center
7401 Holabird Ave., Dundalk, MD 21222
Beck Dunlop, RN 410/955-8795
Susan Davis 410/284-5423/5779

Dystonia Group
Quarterly on Saturdays, 1:30pm
Johns Hopkins Outpatient Center
2nd floor Conference Area, Room 2140
601 North Caroline St., Baltimore MD 21287

Easton/Mid Shore Group
2nd Tuesday of the month, 1:30pm
Talbot Hospice House
586 Cynwood Dr., Easton, MD 21601
Ann Fischer 410/820-2927
Mike O'Neil 410/827-8574

Frederick County Group
3rd Wednesday of the month, 1:00pm
Mt. Pleasant Rurtan Club
8101 Crum Rd., Walkersville, MD 21793
John Kraft 301-845-6514

Hagerstown Group
1st Thursday of the month, 1:30pm
Homewood at Williamsport
16505 Virginia Ave., Williamsport, MD 21795
Peg and Don Barron 301-766-0938

Harford County Group

1st Thursday of the month, 2:00pm
William McFaul Activities Center Multipurpose Room
525 West MacPhail Rd., Bel Air, MD 21014
Beck Dunlop, RN 410/955-8795

Howard County Group

3rd Monday of the month, 7:00pm
Parkinson's & Movement Disorders Center of MD
8180 Lark Brown Rd., Elkridge, MD 21075
Becky Dunlop, RN 410/955-8795

Kensington Exercise and Support Group

Fridays at 10:00am
St. Paul's Methodist Church Heavener Hall
10401 Armory Rd., Kensington, MD 20895
Ed Gessner 301/460-8921
Gaby Rosenberg 301/384-9670

Kensington Carepartner's Group

1st Friday of the month
St. Paul's Methodist Church Heavener Hall
10401 Armory Rd., Kensington, MD 20895
Ann Josseloff 301/946-5468

Laurel Parkinson's Disease Group

Every Tuesday at 10:30am
Laurel Regional Hospital
7300 Van Dusen Rd., Laurel, MD 20707
Sally Heckendom 301-776-3426

LeisureWorld Group

2nd Tuesday of the month, 1:30pm
Leisure World Clubhouse 2
3300 North Leisure World Blvd., Silver Spring, MD 20906
Babs Koch 301-598-7840

Parkinson's Caregiver Group
1st Thursday on the month, 10:00am
Johns Hopkins at Green Spring Station Pavilion II
   (Go through Cafe)
10753 Falls Rd., Lutherville, MD 21093
Becky Dunlop, RN 410/955-8795

Riderwood Group
1st Thursday of the month, 9:30am
Renaissance Building
3128 Gracefield Road, Silver Spring, MD 20904
Molly Bowman, MSW, LGSW 301/572-8496

Southern Maryland Group
4th Saturday of the month
Civista Medical Center Cafeteria
701 East Charles St, LaPlata, MD 20646
Michele Santiago 301-609-4414

University Park Group
4th Thursday of the month, 7:00pm
Riverdale Presbyterian Church Room #1
6513 Queens Chapel Road, University Park, MD 20782
Steve Andrews 301-864-5398

Young Onset/Deep Brain Stimulation Group
Meetings monthly on Saturdays (call for dates), 10:00am
Johns Hopkins Outpatient Center
2nd floor Conference Area, Room 2140
601 North Caroline St., Baltimore MD 21287

The American Parkinson Disease Association, Inc. has a website which lists many chapters for all of the States in this country. There is also a map of the United States where a person can click on a state and all of the information comes right up on the monitor screen. This is very helpful.

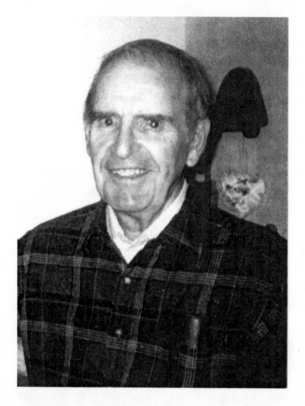

ROBERT FRANCIS AWALT was the second child born to William Joseph Awalt and Marie Molz in Baltimore, Maryland. He attended All Saints Elementary School graduating from the eighth grade and winning the gold medal for scholarship excellence. He next attended the A course at Baltimore Polytechnic High School graduated and continued on to graduate from The Johns Hopkins University with a Bachelor of Engineering degree when he was nineteen years of age. He joined the Navy during World War II and served on the LSM 373 which took supplies to soldiers in the different war zones. After the war was over, Bob Awalt went to work at the Baltimore Gas & Electric Company in Baltimore for almost forty years. During this period of time he returned to Johns Hopkins University to earn a Certificate in Industrial Supervision and Management. He taught in The Johns Hopkins University School of Engineering for more than twenty years. He retired in 1986 to enjoy hobbies and travel.

184

About the Author

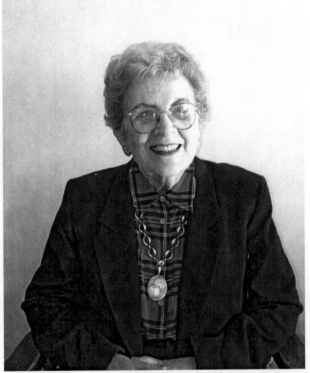

Photo courtesy, Thomas R. Foster

The author was a stay-at-home mom, taking care of two children. She volunteered at schools, libraries, and historical societies. She volunteered at the DAR library in Washington, DC, as a docent for many years and assisted the genealogists in verifying supplemental papers for their members. She and her husband worked at the Baltimore County Historical Society for eight years assisting patrons with genealogy research. She and her husband indexed five ledgers from the old St. James Church in Baltimore for the Catholic Archives. These books were published and given to libraries for researchers. She also completed three years of applications for membership in the patriotic organization Daughters of Colonial Wars. She has researched many lines in her and her husband's family—one line was documented as going back to Charlemagne. She also documented thirty lines of her ancestors arriving in Virginia before 1700. She likes putting clothes on her ancestors' bones.

Printed in the United States
108660LV00001BF/151-498/P